REAL FOOD

FOR

GESTATIONAL

DIABETES

An effective alternative to the
conventional nutrition approach

By

Lily Nichols, RDN, CDE, CLT

Real Food for Gestational Diabetes

www.RealFoodforGD.com

ISBN 13: 978-0-9862950-0-3

Real Food for Gestational Diabetes is intended solely for informational and educational purposes and not as personal medical advice. Always seek the advice of your physician with any questions you have regarding a medical condition, and before undertaking any diet, exercise, or other health program.

The information in this book is not intended to treat, diagnose, cure, or prevent any disease. The approach proposed in this book is not sponsored, approved, recommended, or endorsed by the FDA, USDA, NIH, ADA, AHA, AND, or any other organization.

The author accepts no liability of any kind for any damages caused or alleged to be caused, directly or indirectly, from use of the information in this book.

Cover Design: Lily Nichols
Photography/Graphic Design: Lily Nichols
Layout & Formatting: Sriteja Reddy

Printed in USA

I

Gratitude

Like any book, this would not have been made possible without the help of many people. I thank my colleagues, friends, and family for reviewing the manuscript and otherwise supporting my work.

I'm forever grateful to my colleagues and patients from the California Diabetes and Pregnancy Program: Sweet Success, Harbor UCLA's Women's Health and Perinatal Group, LABioMed, and LA County USC Medical Center. Without your influence, especially that of Dr. Siri Kjos, I would never have developed such a passion for gestational diabetes.

I also extend my appreciation to the women I interviewed for this book who bravely and honestly share their stories – the triumphs and challenges – about managing diabetes during pregnancy.

I thank the loyal readers of my blog, PilatesNutritionist.com, for helping me maintain a consistent practice of writing. You've taught me that my love for real food and prenatal nutrition deserves a larger audience.

Finally, I thank YOU, the reader, for taking the initiative to manage your gestational diabetes and nourish your baby with real food. You have the power to, very literally, change the health of the next generation. This book is, most of all, for you and your baby.

For more information, visit **www.RealFoodforGD.com.**

Table of Contents

Introduction

"They must have done the test wrong. This is a mistake. My doctor is wrong."

Hearing the news that you've been diagnosed with gestational diabetes is hard to swallow.

But not knowing what to do about it is even scarier.

I know because I've worked directly with hundreds of expecting moms with this diagnosis. At first, it feels hopeless.

With the wrong information or no information at all, far too many women struggle with erratic blood sugar, feeling deprived, excessive weight gain, high doses of insulin and medication, and difficult births. Sadly, this often happens while these moms dutifully follow the dietary advice given to them by well-meaning clinicians; a diet that leaves them feeling unsatisfied, unhappy, and confused about ever-increasing blood sugars.

I have also seen the other side of the story. Moms who learn how food affects their blood sugar, who are in tune with their bodies and who know the truth about healthy foods. These moms have a much easier time with their pregnancies. They effortlessly gain the right amount of weight during pregnancy, easily manage their blood sugars, often without medication and insulin, and give birth to beautifully healthy babies.

Having worked as the prenatal nutritionist and diabetes educator under one of the field's most respected perinatologists and consulted for two major gestational diabetes organizations in the United States, I know you can have gestational diabetes *and still* have a healthy baby.

Research has shown us that moms who can bring their blood sugars down to normal have no higher risk of complications than women without the diagnosis. With the right information, gestational diabetes isn't such a bummer after all.

Gestational diabetes gives you a reason to put your self care on the top of the priority list and offers a chance to learn more about nutrition than most people learn in their lifetime. With this book, you have the tools to turn this diagnosis into a blessing in disguise.

This book is for you if you:

- Love food and don't want to be stuck counting calories or following a restrictive meal plan
- Believe your health is your number one priority while pregnant and know that by taking control of your health, you're ensuring the health of your baby
- Want to control your blood sugar without having to rely on insulin or medication (Only your doctor can determine if you need medication; however, good nutrition can help you minimize or avoid it.)

If any of the above ring true for you, then keep reading. The information in this book could very well change your pregnancy, change your life, and change your baby's life.

Chapter 1

What is Gestational Diabetes?

Simply put, gestational diabetes (GD) means that a woman has elevated blood sugar during pregnancy. There are essentially two ways to define it:

Definition 1: Gestational diabetes is a type of diabetes that develops during pregnancy.

Definition 2: Gestational diabetes is a type of diabetes that is *first diagnosed* during pregnancy.

These sound like the same thing, so let me explain how research is challenging our assumptions about this condition.

Definition 1 implies that gestational diabetes is a phenomenon of pregnancy. And in some ways, it is. There are many metabolic changes that occur as a your body adapts to being pregnant that make it difficult to maintain normal blood sugar. Aside from weight gain, there are hormones secreted from the placenta that interfere with the action of insulin (insulin's job to is to lower blood sugar), and insulin resistance goes up (which means your body is less responsive to insulin). All pregnant women are affected by this, but in a woman who develops gestational diabetes, her body is unable to maintain normal blood sugar without changes in diet, exercise, or in some cases, the addition of medication. This particular definition implies that once the mom gives birth, the diabetes goes away. And that's only partially true.

We now know that women diagnosed with gestational diabetes have a high chance of developing prediabetes or type 2 diabetes later in their lifetimes. Within 5 years of delivery, up to 70% of women with gestational diabetes will develop type 2 diabetes.[1] So, in essence, gestational diabetes is the earliest sign that a woman has a predisposition for diabetes.

Definition 2 accounts for women who may have had elevated blood sugar *before* becoming pregnant. By this definition, it's not just the metabolic changes of pregnancy that result in elevated blood sugar, but a woman's state of health before conception. A large portion of the population has undiagnosed prediabetes or type 2 diabetes. Perhaps that explains why GD is, by far, the most common complication of pregnancy, affecting up to 18% of pregnancies.[2] It's estimated that 41% to 53% of GD can be attributed to overweight and obesity.[3]

Of course, weight is not the only player in gestational diabetes, so in the next section, we'll review some of the other risk factors so you can understand this diagnosis better.

Why Me?

One of the first questions I get asked by women is: Why did *I* get diagnosed with gestational diabetes?

Like any other health condition, we will never know for sure what *caused* it, but knowing the risk factors can help you make sense of this.

Risk factors for gestational diabetes:
- Family history of gestational diabetes, prediabetes, or type 2 diabetes
- Overweight at conception
- Age 25 years or older
- Non-Caucasian
- Previous large baby (>8lb. 13oz.), unexplained stillbirth, or malformed infant

Essentially, *everything* is a risk factor for gestational diabetes. Unless you're a thin 23-year-old white woman, you're at risk. But before you start beating yourself up because you 'could've done this or that', know this: up to 50% of women with gestational diabetes have *no risk factors at all.*[4] Even if you *do* have some of the risk factors, not all are within your control. You can't rewind the clock and you can't change your family medical history, but starting now, you *can* make different decisions about food and exercise that will ensure you have a healthy baby.

This sounds like a lot, right? Don't worry. I'll show you how to change your diet and choose the right exercise in the upcoming chapters.

Why is Maintaining Normal Blood Sugar So Important?

Your doctor has already explained that gestational diabetes means your blood sugar is higher than it should be during pregnancy. Sometimes it's hard to understand why having slightly elevated blood sugar is a big deal. I mean, it's *just sugar*, right?

It turns out the level of sugar in your bloodstream is *really* important, especially while pregnant. Having elevated blood sugar can lead to the following problems:

- Birth defects
- Large babies (also called macrosomia)
- Birth injury – Shoulders of large babies can dislocate or become stuck during vaginal delivery (also called shoulder distocia). This may lead to neurological damage to the infant or a medical emergency for the mom.
- Hypoglycemia – baby's blood sugar is too low at birth
- Jaundice
- Higher rates of C-sections
- Higher risk of preeclampsia (pregnancy-induced high blood pressure that poses a risk to mother and baby)
- Permanent changes to a child's metabolism - Elevated blood sugar can "turn on" the genes that predispose your infant to obesity, diabetes, and heart disease in their lifetime.

In fact, children exposed to gestational diabetes in the womb have a 6-fold higher risk of blood sugar problems at adolescence, including impaired glucose tolerance and type 2 diabetes.[5] However, we know moms who maintain good blood sugar control throughout their pregnancies lessen these risks. Truly, health starts *in utero*!

Summary

As you can see, the risks associated with gestational diabetes are real, so there's no time like the present to learn how to control your blood sugar and make this a happy, healthy pregnancy.

I'll be right here with you to explain everything, both in this book and over at **www.RealFoodforGD.com**. There's a lot to learn, but it's really not too complicated. I promise!

Emily's Story

When I received the call from the nurse and heard the words I was dreading: "You have gestational diabetes", I remember feeling devastated; like my whole dream of a vaginal birth after C-section (VBAC) just got flushed down the toilet in the blink of an eye. I felt like a failure. Since the moment I found out I was pregnant, I had immediately started a lower carb and lower sugar diet, hoping to avoid GD, as I was told I had borderline GD during my first pregnancy, and knew that with my older "advanced maternal age" of 36, I'd be at higher risk this time around. I didn't understand why, if I had taken all of these precautions to avoid GD, my body was failing me despite my efforts.

For about three days after I got the news, I was very scared. I went through the motions of learning how to test my sugars and felt a slight sense of hope when my fasting sugars were all under control in the mornings. From my research, I knew that if I could avoid medications, this would be a good thing all around. I kept on my low carb and low sugar diet and began spending my nights researching online as much as I could about GD and how to control it.

The first important thing I learned was that GD was not something I caused, but rather was something having to do with the way my placenta processed sugars and hindered the effectiveness of the insulin in my body. This was a great relief, and helped me feel less guilty and less like my body failed me. I joined a number of Facebook and online groups and reached out for support around this issue, which really helped.

With all of the information I read and the support I was getting, I began to feel more in control of the situation, and decided that I would do everything I could to control the GD with diet and exercise. I knew that eating a small meal or snack every 2 hours was important to keep my sugars in check. My midwife said that I could meet with a nutritionist if I wanted to, but if I felt informed enough, I didn't have to. I looked up general carb intake guidelines online, and was surprised at how high the recommendations generally seemed to be. Even the celebrated Brewers diet seemed excessive to me.

My general philosophy, I decided, was to eat as healthy a diet as possible, keep portions in check, eat every two hours, cheat every once in a while, and make sure I knew what types of food spiked my sugars (and adjust my diet accordingly). I decided I didn't feel I needed to meet with someone so they could tell me how and what to eat, as my blood glucose monitor would give me the feedback I needed, and I could listen to my body and keep track of how food was affecting my energy levels/etc. I walked my dog almost every day, for at least 30 minutes, as briskly as possible, and drank a ton of water.

Throughout the pregnancy I monitored my weight gain, and was surprised that though my belly was growing (and measured perfectly at each prenatal appointment), the rest of me was not blowing up or swelling. I kept getting compliments about how great I looked and how I was "all belly"; I am only 5 feet, and was 134 when I got pregnant, so weight does easily show on my small frame. Though it was great to get all of the positive feedback, the best part about the small weight gain was how great I felt physically. During my first pregnancy (during which I gained 25 lbs), I remember feeling quite heavy, weighed down, and had swelling in my fingers and feet. I remember developing a "double chin" at the end of my pregnancy and feeling so unattractive! I also felt much more tired and sluggish.

With the low carb and low sugar diet, I only gained a total of 12 pounds the entire pregnancy. My midwife was happy with the way I was controlling my sugars with diet and exercise, and did not make a fuss about the GD. This boosted my confidence, and helped me stay on track emotionally and psychologically to try for the VBAC.

On August 8th, I gave birth to a perfectly healthy 7 lb, 3 ounce baby boy. The birth was a smooth, uncomplicated and successful VBAC. Though I was initially devastated that I had GD with this pregnancy, looking back, it was actually quite a

8

blessing: The low carb and low sugar diet actually kept me on track in terms of my nutrition and my eating, it kept my weight gain in check, it might have kept my baby's weight gain in check and most importantly, it kept both my baby and me as healthy as possible.

Though I am fairly certain I am done having children, if I were to become pregnant again, I would no doubt follow this diet and this philosophy again, regardless of whether or not I had a GD diagnosis. I hope this story helps someone have the birth and the healthy child they desire!

Chapter 2

What Now? What Can I Do?

Have you heard the saying "knowledge is power"?

When it comes to your health and your pregnancy, nothing could ring more true. Yes, the diagnosis of gestational diabetes can come as a surprise, and yes, it can be frustrating. But understanding what is happening in your body gives you the power to influence your blood sugar and ultimately, the trajectory of your pregnancy and the health of your baby.

So what are we waiting for? Let's dive right in!

Understanding What's Going on in Your Body

Gestational diabetes is actually treated similarly to prediabetes or type 2 diabetes. Why? Because it's essentially the same thing: insulin resistance. In the case of gestational diabetes, insulin resistance was first identified during your pregnancy, but as I discussed in Chapter 1, it could have been going on before you got pregnant (undiagnosed prediabetes). Either way, how you manage it is the same.

What is Insulin Resistance?

Insulin is a hormone released from your pancreas that helps remove sugar from your bloodstream and deliver it to your cells to be used as energy. When you have insulin resistance, your body stops responding normally to insulin. When the blood sugar is consistently elevated, the pancreas is forced to release high amounts of insulin, quite frequently, in order to keep the blood sugar within normal levels.

After a while, your body becomes so accustomed to high levels of insulin that it stops responding to it. It's like that annoying neighbor who *always* knocks on your door. After a while, you start to ignore your neighbor and forget she's even knocking. This means you can have high blood sugar *and* high insulin, but insulin is no longer able to perform its job. In other words, your cells have become *resistant* to the actions of insulin.

Pregnancy, even without gestational diabetes, naturally induces insulin resistance. Why? Because humans evolved with famine and periods of starvation where food, especially food rich in carbohydrates, was scarce. Insulin resistance meant that a mom's body would not take too much energy and instead divert those nutrients to the growing baby. It's a built-in (and actually, quite brilliant) mechanism for survival.

But now that we live in a world with abundant food and carbohydrates, this natural adaptation works against us. Is starving yourself the solution? Absolutely not! But choosing foods that naturally *don't* raise the blood sugar very much while avoiding foods that spike the blood sugar is the obvious and most rational solution. We'll delve into that topic in Chapter 3.

As your pregnancy progresses and your body releases ever increasing amounts of hormones (estrogen, progesterone, cortisol, and human placental lactogen), insulin resistance gets worse. This is part of the reason why gestational diabetes tends to be screened for and diagnosed in the end of the second trimester (between 24-28 weeks).

This also explains why women are more likely to need the help of blood sugar-lowering medication or insulin shots during the third trimester to keep their blood sugar at normal levels (though many can still do this with diet and exercise alone). With more undiagnosed prediabetes being seen in pregnant women, some providers screen during the first trimester with a test called A1c (hemoglobin A1c). This measures your average blood sugar over 3 months and if it's higher than normal (5.7% or greater), you may be diagnosed with gestational diabetes.

However it was diagnosed, what matters now is to pay attention to your blood sugar levels so you can learn how to keep them at normal levels.

Checking Your Blood Sugar

The best way to learn about your blood sugar (also called blood glucose) is to test it at home. Your blood sugar changes throughout the day for a variety of reasons and no two women's blood sugar patterns are the same. Testing your blood sugar regularly at home will help you understand what makes your blood sugar come out high or low, which is crucial to proactively managing your gestational diabetes.

Your healthcare provider may provide you with a blood glucose meter (also called a glucometer) and the test strips to begin monitoring at home. Or, you may purchase these supplies from a pharmacy, even without a prescription.

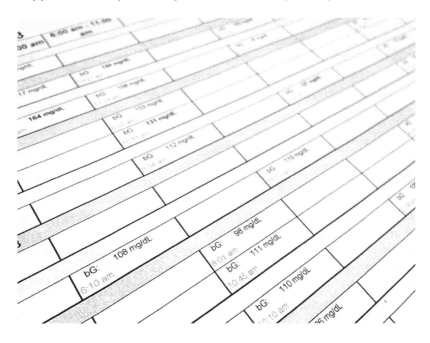

What is Normal Blood Sugar? What's Too High? What's Too Low?

If you have relatives who have diabetes, you might be familiar with what's considered normal, high, or low blood sugar. However, during pregnancy the normal levels for blood sugar are slightly lower compared to non-pregnant adults.

Part of this is because pregnant women have more diluted blood, since pregnancy increases fluid in the circulatory system by at least a liter. This extra fluid dilutes the blood sugar. So be sure to use the below guidelines or those given to you by your medical provider, *not* what your non-pregnant family members with diabetes are using.

Blood Sugar Goals During Pregnancy

The standards for "normal" blood sugar during pregnancy have changed over the years, mostly in response to recent research that has shown even mildly elevated blood sugar can leave permanent effects on a child's metabolism. That has led a number of organizations, including the progressive California Diabetes and Pregnancy Program, to lower the goals for fasting blood sugar from 95mg/dl down to 90mg/dl. These target blood sugar values may very well decrease in the future, as I'll explain below.

Fasting Blood Sugar

This blood sugar reading is taken first thing in the morning before any foods or caloric beverages are consumed. Normal fasting blood sugar in pregnancy is less than or equal to 90mg/dl. Blood sugar measured immediately *before* eating a meal should also be close to or less than 90mg/dl, although before-meal blood sugar is less commonly monitored.

Post-Meal Blood Sugar

This blood sugar reading is taken 1-2 hours after the *first bite* of food. Generally, this number should be less than or equal to 130mg/dl. The longer you wait to check your blood sugar after eating, the lower the number should be. Many specialists suggest post-meal blood sugar should be less than 120mg/dl, particularly if you check 2 hours after eating. I personally suggest aiming for less than 120mg/dl after meals.

Blood sugar levels significantly higher than the above values can be dangerous for your baby. Blood sugars consistently higher than 140mg/dl after meals may mean your baby will be large at delivery, also called macrosomia. When this becomes a pattern, the baby will begin over-producing its own insulin to try to lower the blood sugar, essentially wearing out its little pancreas before he or she is ever born. The combination of high insulin and high blood sugar signals the baby to accumulate more fat than normal. This predisposes your baby to obesity and diabetes later in life (and life-threatening hypoglycemia at birth).[6]

Blood sugars beyond 200mg/dl are particularly harmful, and have been linked to heart defects, missing limbs, and other structural deformities in infants. However, these risks are generally seen in women with undiagnosed type 2 diabetes or poorly controlled type 1 diabetes who experience uncontrolled blood sugars during the *first 8 weeks* of pregnancy, when organs are forming. High blood sugars experienced in later pregnancy are linked to stillbirth and macrosomia. If your blood sugar is nearing those levels, call your doctor or medical provider immediately.

When is Blood Sugar Too Low?

Since pregnancy naturally induces lower blood sugar, the cutoff for low blood sugar (also called hypoglycemia) is also lower compared to non-pregnant adults. Hypoglycemia in pregnancy is blood sugar less than 60mg/dl. If your blood sugar is below 60mg/dl, it may mean you haven't eaten in a while. If you're taking medication/insulin, it might also mean that you need an adjustment in dosage, timing, exercise, or meal/snack timing or composition.

In my experience, true hypoglycemia is rare in pregnant women not taking medication or insulin, but if you get any symptoms of low blood sugar, check your blood sugar immediately. Symptoms include hunger, nausea, sweating or clammy skin, anxiety, nervousness, increased heart rate, mood changes, and low energy. If your blood sugar is below 60mg/dl, eat a snack or meal that contains some carbohydrates and re-test your blood sugar 15 minutes later to ensure it has increased. One of the "moderate carb snacks" listed in Chapter 4 is a good choice in this situation.

Average Blood Sugar in Pregnant Women

While the above guidelines are useful, some doctors have begun suggesting lower blood sugar targets be adopted. This is in response to research showing that fetal macrosomia (big babies) are common even in women who meet these targets.

"Even when current glucose targets are achieved in the pregnancy affected by diabetes, macrosomia still occurs and *in utero* programming may have a lasting metabolic impact on the offspring."[6]

Healthy weight pregnant women without gestational diabetes have the following average blood sugars:

- Fasting: 70.9 ± 7.8 mg/dl
- One Hour Post-Meal: 108.9 ± 12.9 mg/dl
- Two Hours Post-Meal: 99.3 ±10.2 mg/dl

The 24 hour average blood sugar in healthy pregnant women ranges from 77.4 ± 4.7 to 97 ± 9 mg/dL. We know that the closer you are to "normal" blood sugar, the healthier your pregnancy and the healthier your baby. I suggest discussing your target blood sugar with your doctor.

How Often Should I Check?

Most experts suggest checking your blood sugar four times per day:
- Fasting
- 1-2 hours after breakfast
- 1-2 hours after lunch

- 1-2 hours after dinner

Some doctors may also have you check your blood sugar before meals if you require insulin or medication to manage them (occasionally, you may be asked to check your blood sugar in the middle of the night). In general, unless a woman is taking insulin/medication, blood sugar is checked to ensure it is not too high.

Tips For Checking Your Blood Sugar

- Wash your hands in warm, soapy water before checking
- Avoid the use of lotions immediately before checking your blood sugar, as these may give false highs
- Make sure your meter is calibrated (see manufacturer instructions)
- Double check that testing strips are not expired or have been opened too long/stored improperly
- Use a clean lancet (the needle used to prick your finger to get a drop of blood). In general, do not reuse a lancet more than 3 times. If sharing a lancing device with a family member, use a new lancet *every* time you check your blood sugar.
- Prick the side of your finger, not the tip or center, since the sides have fewer nerve endings and better blood flow.
- Regularly switch fingers to avoid calluses and scarring.

Keeping Track of Blood Sugars

Before making any changes to your usual eating habits and routine, it's helpful to begin monitoring your blood sugar and observe the results to make a baseline assessment. Most meters store data for later use, but I find writing down the blood sugar values along with your food intake, exercise, and other factors (stress, energy levels, hunger/fullness, etc.), can be very educational.

Every body is different, and while there are some usual culprits for high or low blood sugar, only *you* can identify your unique response to food, exercise, and other factors. Also, if you run into any difficulty figuring out why you have blood sugar numbers outside the normal range, you can bring this detailed log to your healthcare practitioner for guidance.

At the end of this chapter, you'll find a sample Food & Blood Sugar Log to begin monitoring.

What's Next?

Now that you understand what's going on inside your body and how to monitor your blood sugar, let's delve in to the primary way you'll be managing gestational diabetes: real food!

FOOD & BLOOD SUGAR LOG (EXAMPLE)

Date	BG	Breakfast	BG	Lunch	BG	Dinner	BG	Bedtime Snack
Mon	85	2 eggs over-easy, butter 1 slice whole wheat bread 1 cup black tea + cream ✓ 30 min walk, moderate pace	105	2 chicken thighs Salad: lettuce, kale, tomato, avocado, balsamic vinaigrette, 1 chocolate chip cookie ✗ 1/2 banana	125	Meatloaf, roasted cauliflower, bell peppers, and onions 1 cup blueberries with whipped cream (unsweetened)	94	1/2 cup Greek yogurt + pecans
Tues	88	2 eggs over-easy, butter 1 slice whole wheat bread 1 cup black tea + cream	115	4 oz carnitas 1 small corn tortilla Tomato salsa, sour cream Bell peppers, onions, lettuce	94	Roasted chicken 1/2 cup lentils Sautéed zucchini and onions ✓ 30 min walk, moderate pace	102	2 oz cheese + 6 whole grain crackers
Wed	87	1 cup cottage cheese 1/2 cup chopped fresh fruit small handful pecans ✓ Pilates class (60 min)	98	2 slices pizza ✗ Salad with balsamic	138	Lettuce-wrapped burger Cheese, tomato, lettuce, pickles, mustard 1 Tbsp ketchup	99	no snack- oops! ✗
Thurs	96							
Fri								
Sat								
Sun								

BG= blood glucose   ✓ Track exercise (type, duration, intensity)   ✗ Mark food(s) suspected of causing high blood sugar

19

FOOD & BLOOD SUGAR LOG

Date	BG	Breakfast	BG	Lunch	BG	Dinner	BG	Bedtime Snack
Mon								
Tues								
Wed								
Thurs								
Fri								
Sat								
Sun								

BG= blood glucose   ✔ Track exercise (type, duration, intensity)   ✗ Mark food(s) suspected of causing high blood sugar

20

Sara's Story

When I got diagnosed with gestational diabetes at 29 weeks, it was all a whirlwind. They tell you a diagnosis, they bring you a prescription, and then they bring you a box of needles, a meter, and tell you to take your blood sugar. Before you even know what's going on, your world completely changes.

Luckily I was referred to a gestational diabetes class, but I had to wait *5 days* to see the dietitian! In the interim I was left wondering what all these numbers meant and what I should do about it. That's when I really started to worry about all the risks. I had always had large babies (three of them were over 9 pounds), but no gestational diabetes. This time, with my fifth pregnancy, I got the diagnosis. So was I doomed to have an *even bigger* baby this time?!

When I saw the dietitian, it was so far from how I eat; she had all these packages of pre-prepared meals and so many processed carbohydrates. They told me to eat a high-carbohydrate diet - eating carbs at breakfast - lunch - dinner - and 3 snacks per day. I was instructed to limit my fat intake as much as possible.

I started eating low carb before I got pregnant because I struggled with fertility. I started Atkins and within a month of starting that diet, I got pregnant. I had a hard time understanding why I needed a whopping 200g of carbohydrates per day because everything I had learned about nutrition before this had me believe I should limit carbohydrates. I tried the diet for a little while, but this level of carbs was just too much for me, and my blood sugar numbers after meals were way too high.

So I decided that during my pregnancy, I'd keep my carbohydrates between 75-100g per day (higher than what I ate before I conceived, but still nowhere near the "recommended" amount). My numbers were fine except for my fasting numbers in the morning unless I had a snack in the middle of the night. I tried a lot to get my fasting blood sugar under control, but I ended up needing glyburide at night to lower them.

It was a pretty lonely road, since there were few low carb pregnancy support groups and so many unanswered questions. Luckily my doctor was supportive of my decision to stay low carb while pregnant and she could see the positive impact it was having on my pregnancy. It seemed like most other doctors just told women to up their carbs and up their medication, but I was fortunate to not have this experience.

Funny enough, my 5th child, despite me having gestational diabetes, was born weighing 8 pounds 3 ounces, which is small for me! I believe eating low carb helped my health and my baby's immensely.

Looking back, I had all the risk factors for GD. I was overweight, my mom had gestational diabetes when pregnant with me (and has type 2 diabetes now), I was over 35, and 3 of my children were big at birth. And, even though it was scary at first, the diagnosis turned out to be a good thing, because it made me realize how much my health is related to what I eat.

Having gestational diabetes changed not only my eating, but how I feed my kids. My kids now gravitate towards foods that aren't processed carbohydrates. They've been raised in a household without those foods and all of them are at a healthy weight. I'm a better mom and a better example to all of my children because of gestational diabetes.

Chapter 3

Nutrition for Gestational Diabetes

In the first chapter I gave you two definitions of gestational diabetes. But there is an alternative and more telling description of this diagnosis: carbohydrate intolerance during pregnancy.

Why do I say this? Because this shifts the focus from the problem, high blood sugar, to the solution, a diet limited in carbohydrates.

Maybe you were referred to a dietitian, or maybe you've heard nothing about what to eat for GD. This chapter will give you the tools to choose the healthiest foods for you and baby that will keep your blood sugar under control naturally.

How Food Affects Your Blood Sugar

The first step in controlling your blood sugar is understanding how food affects it. Many dietitians and diabetes educators will try to complicate the explanation, but I like to keep things simple. Let's start from the top.

We get energy from three macronutrients: carbohydrates, fat, and protein.

Each of these nutrients has a different impact on your blood sugar levels. We'll begin by talking about the foods that affect blood sugar the most, carbohydrates. Then we'll look at all the foods that *don't* raise the blood sugar. Rest assured, there are a lot of 'em!

Foods That Raise Your Blood Sugar

Carbohydrates

Carbohydrates are the *only* macronutrient that significantly raises the blood sugar. For this reason, carbohydrates are the *only* nutrient we need to watch closely in women who have gestational diabetes. Carbohydrates are like long chains of sugar all linked together. When we digest them, our body breaks them down into individual chain links of sugar to absorb them. Once the sugar is absorbed, your blood sugar level goes up.

With that in mind, when learning about what combinations of food work best for your body, you'll want to know which foods are highest in carbohydrates:

- Grains: whole grains, refined grains, and anything made with flour (e.g., pasta, bread, tortillas, pancakes, crackers, cereals, granola)
- Legumes: beans, lentils, split peas
- Starchy Vegetables: potatoes, sweet potatoes/yams, winter squash, peas, corn
- Fruit
- Milk and Yogurt

If you're nutrition savvy, you may notice that some of the above foods are also good sources of protein and wonder why are they counted as a carbohydrate. Well, although legumes, peas, milk, and yogurt all contain protein, they also contain high levels of carbohydrate and therefore significantly contribute to high blood sugar levels.

For that reason, they are counted in the carbohydrate group. They are, however, a wise carbohydrate choice compared to breads, crackers, pasta, and cereals because of their protein content. Legumes are also rich in fiber, which slows how quickly the carbohydrates are digested. Since these high-fiber examples slowly raise the blood sugar, you may hear people describe them as having a "low glycemic index."

The above list does not include *all* sources of carbohydrates in the diet, just the ones with the highest concentrations compared to other whole foods. Carbohydrates are found in many other real foods, but in smaller proportions in relation to other nutrients. These would include nuts, seeds, non-starchy vegetables, and a few others. However, these foods have a low glycemic index, because they are also a source of fiber, fat, and/or protein. Unless your blood sugar is still high after accounting for the carbohydrate-rich foods listed above, you can eat nuts, seeds, and non-starchy vegetables freely without worrying.

Carbohydrate Portions

It's helpful to measure your portions of carbohydrate foods so you can better understand how they affect your blood sugar. For simplicity, diabetes educators will often suggest measuring carbohydrates in "portions." One "portion" of carbohydrates is equal to 15 grams of carbohydrate, and the volume of food that contains 15 grams of carbohydrate varies considerably, as you'll see below.

One "portion" or 15 grams of carbohydrates is equivalent to:
- 1 slice of bread (white or whole grain)
- 1 small corn tortilla
- ½ cup of cereal (varies product to product)
- ½ cup cooked pasta
- ½ cup cooked rice, oatmeal, or other grain
- ½ cup beans
- ½ cup sweet potatoes, white potatoes, corn, peas, or other starchy vegetable

You'll notice with grains and starches that approximately half a cup is a serving. With other foods, the serving sizes may be larger.
- 1 cup milk
- 1 cup plain yogurt
- ½ cup fresh fruit (or a baseball-sized piece of fruit)
- ½ large banana
- 1 cup berries

For comparison, you could eat 2 cups of non-starchy vegetables (such as broccoli, cauliflower, zucchini, etc) to equal the carbohydrates in only ½ cup of cooked rice; or 10 cups of green, leafy vegetables (lettuce, spinach, kale, etc.)!

Counting Carbohydrates

You can use food labels to more accurately identify the amount of carbohydrates in a particular food. The "total carbohydrate" count on labels accounts for the sugar, fiber, and other carbohydrates in a specified amount of that food. Because fiber does not raise the blood sugar, some people calculate "net carbohydrates", which is the total grams of carbohydrate minus the grams of fiber, to better estimate how much their blood sugar will be impacted by eating that food.

Some processed foods are very concentrated in carbohydrates and are best limited or avoided completely. In my personal experience, women experience the best blood sugar control (and maximize their nutrient intake) by getting most of their carbohydrates from non-starchy foods.

If you've been told to eat more carbohydrates to avoid ketosis (and maybe you're not even sure what that means), be sure to read Chapter 11.

Now that you understand where carbohydrates are found in your diet, let's move on to the foods that don't contain many carbohydrates.

Nutrition Facts

Serving Size 1/2 cup (57g)
Servings Per Container 10

Amount Per Serving

Calories 190   Calories from Fat 25

%**Daily Value***

Total Fat 3g	**5%**
Saturated Fat 1g	**5%**
Trans Fat 0g	
Cholesterol 0mg	**0%**
Sodium 95mg	**4%**
Total Carbohydrate 38g	**13%**
Dietary Fiber 5g	**20%**
Sugars 3g	
Protein 2g	

Vitamin A 0%	•	Vitamin C 0%	
Calcium 4%	•	Iron 6%	

* Percent Daily Values are based on a 2,000 calorie diet. Your Daily Values may be higher or lower depending on your calorie needs:

	Calories:	2,000	2,500
Total Fat	Less than	65g	80g
Sat Fat	Less than	20g	25g
Cholesterol	Less than	300mg	300mg
Sodium	Less than	2,400mg	2,400mg
Total Carb		300g	375g
Dietary Fiber		25g	30g

The company's serving size is ½ cup. All nutrients below reflect the amount in ½ cup.

½ cup contains 38g of carbohydrate in total. Of those 38g, 5g come from fiber & 3g come from sugar.

If you subtract the fiber, this product has *33g of net carbs*.

If you eat ½ cup, you are eating approx. 2 carbohydrate servings.

Although this food is high in fiber, it's high in carbs, low in protein, and low in fat. This food would likely spike your blood sugar.

27

Foods That DON'T Raise Your Blood Sugar

Vegetables

Aside from the high-carbohydrate vegetables mentioned above (potatoes, sweet potatoes/yams, winter squash, peas, corn), most vegetables have little effect on the blood sugar. As a whole, these are referred to as non-starchy vegetables and they should make up the bulk of your vegetable intake (and actually, the bulk of your diet).

Most of the carbohydrates in non-starchy vegetables come from fiber, which does not get converted into sugar in large quantities. Fiber also tends to slow down how quickly your body breaks down other carbohydrates and converts them into sugar (similar to the way fat and protein work).

Below is a list of non-starchy vegetables. Towards the bottom of the list, I use an asterisk to mark what I consider to be moderately-starchy vegetables. If you are very sensitive to carbohydrates, you may need to watch your portions of these. In general though, unless you're eating more than 1 cup at a sitting or are drinking vegetable juice, moderately-starchy vegetables are unlikely to significantly raise your blood sugar. I give you the distinction below in case you need to fine-tune your diet to achieve normal blood sugar after meals.

I suggest eating non-starchy vegetables to satiety (that feeling of having enough to be satisfied, but not overstuffed), without worrying about portion size.

Non-Starchy Vegetables:
- artichoke
- asparagus
- bell pepper
- broccoli
- Brussels sprouts
- cabbage
- cactus

- cauliflower
- celery
- chayote squash
- cilantro/parsley
- cucumber
- eggplant
- garlic
- greens: beet, collard, dandelion, mustard, spinach, kale, chard, turnip greens, spinach,watercress, bok choy
- tomatillo
- tomato
- green beans
- kohlrabi
- leek
- lettuce: endive, escarole, iceberg, romaine, "baby" greens
- mushroom
- okra
- onion (all types)
- radish
- rutabaga
- summer squash
- zucchini
- beet*
- carrot*
- jicama*
- parsnip*
- snap peas, snow peas*
- spaghetti squash*
- turnip*

*Moderately-starchy vegetables: These vegetables have up to 15g net carbs per cup.

Fats & Proteins

Foods that are primarily composed of fat and protein *don't* raise the blood sugar, at least not directly. Rather, they stabilize the blood sugar, both preventing it from going too high or too low. Similar to non-starchy vegetables, I suggest eating protein and fat to satiety without worrying about portion size.

Generally speaking, pregnant women benefit from a *minimum* of 80g of protein per day, which is easily met if you include small portions of protein-rich foods at each meal and snack.

When reducing carbohydrates in your diet, it's important that you still consume enough calories to provide your body (and your baby) with sufficient energy. For that reason, and others which I'll explore in later chapters, I do *not* suggest limiting your intake of fat from real food. In fact, you may benefit from increasing it.

Foods that are rich in fat and protein are listed below.

Meats:
- Beef, lamb, pork, buffalo, etc. (ideally from pasture-raised animals)
- Poultry (ideally from pasture-raised animals)
- Fish & Seafood (ideally wild-caught)
- Sausage & bacon (ideally from pasture-raised animals)
- Homemade bone broth or stock

Eggs & Dairy:
- Eggs (ideally from pasture-raised chickens)
- Cheese - all types (cheddar, mozzarella, etc.), cream cheese, cottage cheese*, ricotta cheese, paneer
- Plain Greek yogurt*
- Heavy whipping cream, sour cream, labne
- Butter

Nuts/Seeds*:
- Almonds, pecans, peanuts, walnuts, hazelnuts, pumpkin seeds, sunflower seeds, macadamia nuts, cashews, etc.
- Nut butter*, such as peanut butter or almond butter
- Coconut products, including oil, full-fat milk, coconut cream, shredded coconut (The only coconut product to limit is coconut water, which is high in carbohydrates.)
- Chia seeds, flax seeds, sunflower seeds, etc.

Fatty Fruits:
- Avocado*
- Olives

Oils & Fats:
- Animal fats: butter, ghee, lard, tallow, duck fat, etc.
- Plant fats: olive oil, coconut oil, avocado oil, macadamia nut oil, etc. (Choose "extra virgin" oils. Plant oils are easily damaged with heat, so avoid cooking at high temperatures, with the exception of coconut oil.)
    - o *Avoid* processed vegetables oils including: corn oil, soybean oil, canola oil, peanut oil, safflower oil, and cottonseed oil
- Mayonnaise
- Salad dressings (free of added sugars)

*These foods contain small amounts of net carbohydrates, while the other foods in this list contain virtually none.

You'll notice some dairy products included in this list, namely butter, cream, plain Greek yogurt, and cheese. These are not a significant source of carbohydrates, unlike milk and yogurt, so they do not raise the blood sugar significantly. Greek yogurt is strained, which removes most of the lactose (the form of carbohydrate in dairy) and concentrates the protein.

Later chapters will explore the importance of sourcing quality animal foods and seafood. For now, let's stay focused on how these foods affect your blood sugar.

How to Combine Foods

Now that you understand which foods raise the blood sugar and which foods don't, let's see how this would fit into a well balanced meal or snack.

Let's start with a simple example.

Take an apple. If you eat that apple by itself, your blood sugar will go up and it will do so rapidly because apples are high in carbohydrates and have very little fat or protein.

Now, take that same apple, but this time eat it with a small handful of almonds. Your blood sugar will still go up, because there are carbohydrates in the apple, *but* your blood sugar might not go up *as high* or go up *as quickly* because the fat and protein in the almonds will slow down how fast those carbohydrates are digested and absorbed.

I like to think of eating the apple by itself as eating "naked carbohydrates." When you "dress it up" by matching it with another food that contains fat and protein, your body responds completely differently (in a good way). When your blood sugar doesn't spike, it also doesn't crash. That means you stay full for longer and have fewer sugar cravings.

This same approach works when planning meals as well.

The Plate Method

The Plate Method is a great way to visually plan out your meals without strictly measuring portions. Aim for half of your plate to come from non-starchy vegetables, one quarter of your plate from proteins and fats, and the remaining one quarter to come from carbohydrates (generally no more than 1 cup total, or 30 grams of carbohydrates, at one sitting). Some women may need less than 30 grams of carbohydrates per meal to maintain normal blood sugar. See the next chapter for more specific meal advice.

Unlike most dietitians, I shy away from providing strict portion measurements unless your blood sugar is not well controlled with the above guidelines. Only you will be able to determine that by checking your blood sugar 1-2 hours after each meal.

If your blood sugar is elevated above 120mg/dl after a meal, it's likely that you overate carbohydrates and it's a good idea to measure carbohydrate portions in the future. Some like to use measuring cups for the first few weeks until they get used to "eye-balling it." However, other women find it necessary to continue to measure portions or count carbohydrates throughout their pregnancy in order keep their blood sugars controlled.

If you you are hungry within 2 hours after eating a meal, I suggest increasing the quantity of proteins, fats, and non-starchy vegetables in future meals. If your blood sugar remains below 120mg/dl, you could also slightly increase your carbohydrate portions.

Mindful Eating

Some women feel nervous without having strict guidance on portions or calories. One of the most effective and natural ways to ensure you're getting the right amount of food for your body is to apply mindful eating techniques. Mindful eating means listening to the signals your body sends you about food and honoring what it has to say. It means eating when you're hungry and stopping when your body has had enough.

Many times we eat on autopilot, since we've become disconnected from our body's inner cues or perhaps because we're responding only to external cues. Sometimes that means we eat everything on our plate regardless of how full we feel (the "clean your plate" trap). Or we eat simply because everyone around us is eating, even when our body is not hungry for more food. On the other hand, you might feel like you need to restrict your food because you have gestational diabetes and begin to avoid eating even when you're hungry. None of the above is healthy. When we ignore our hunger cues, we ignore our fullness cues as well. So mindlessly overeating or consciously undereating are equally unhealthy and unsustainable.

But our bodies are incredible teachers and they are always communicating with us. It takes practice to tune into these cues, but I promise you that over time, you'll learn to trust your body again. To begin eating more mindfully, try the following Hunger Awareness Exercise.

Hunger Awareness Exercise:

Before each meal or snack, calmly check in with how your body is feeling. Do you have any sensations of hunger? Is there a gnawing feeling in the stomach? Is it mild or intense? Are you hungry for a small amount of food or do you want a whole meal? How are your energy levels? What kinds of foods are you craving - sweet, salty, something else? (This only needs to take 15-30 seconds.)

In the middle of your meal or snack, check in again. Are you starting to feel full? What sensations is your body sending you? Are the flavors and textures of this food satisfying or would you prefer to stop and eat something else? How quickly are you eating - slow, moderate, or fast? Ask these questions without judgement. No answer is right or wrong.

Towards the end of your meal or snack, do a final check in. What would your body say if it could talk? Would it ask for more? Would it tell you to stop eating? Would it tell you that there's absolutely, positively no more room for food? How did your body respond to the speed at which you were eating? Again, ask these questions without judgement. No answer is right or wrong.

You might start to notice patterns in the way you eat. Maybe you rush through meals, or you feel driven to clean your plate even when you're full. Maybe you have anxiety while you eat because you're nervous about how your blood sugar levels will be afterwards.

Ideally, you want to eat until you no longer feel hungry and also do not feel uncomfortably full. If it's helpful, you can add these notes to your Food & Blood Sugar Log and see if your blood sugar numbers are affected. You might be pleasantly surprised to find this approach reduces your cravings, your anxiety around eating, and your blood sugar levels.[7]

Meal Timing & Spacing

With gestational diabetes, it's important to be sure your blood sugar never gets too high or too low. Since we know blood sugar goes up every time you eat (assuming you're eating some foods that contain carbohydrates), it's wise to space small meals and snacks a few hours apart.

Eating in this way ensures:
1. You never get too hungry or let your blood sugar get too low
2. You don't have to eat huge portions, which could spike your blood sugar
3. Your baby gets a consistent supply of nutrients throughout the day

Smaller meals are also helpful if you're managing common pregnancy complaints like morning sickness, nausea or vomiting, heartburn, reflux, or feeling full quickly.

Foods To Avoid

Refined Carbohydrates

You've likely heard the term "refined carbohydrates" before. This refers to low-fiber, processed carbohydrates that digest and absorb rapidly, causing a spike in blood sugar. In other words, these foods have a high glycemic index. They also tend to have low nutrient-density, meaning they are primarily composed of carbohydrates while being low in vitamins, minerals, and antioxidants. These "filler foods" leave less room for more nutrient-dense foods in the diet.

Foods High in Refined Carbohydrates:
- Refined grain products, including anything made from white flour (bread, bagels, pizza, pasta, noodles, crackers, pretzels, chips, etc.)
- Breakfast cereal or "puffed" grains (popcorn, rice cakes)
- "Instant" products, namely instant rice (or quick-cooking rice), instant noodles (like ramen), instant potatoes, and instant oatmeal (or quick oats)
- White rice

- White potatoes

Although potatoes are technically a whole food, they have a very high glycemic index. You may need to avoid or limit your consumption of them to prevent hyperglycemia.

Sugar

It might be obvious to you already, but foods that contain high amounts of sugar (added *or* naturally occurring) are best avoided when you're managing diabetes during pregnancy. If you do choose to include these on occasion, keep your portions small and eat less of other carbohydrate foods with that meal or snack. (For example, if you want ice cream after dinner, have a low-carbohydrate dinner, such as chicken with vegetables instead of pasta.)

Foods High in Sugar:
- Sugar: white sugar, brown sugar, raw sugar, molasses, honey, agave nectar, syrups (like corn syrup, maple syrup, or brown rice syrup), date sugar, coconut sugar, sucrose, dextrose, fructose, maltose, etc.
- Sweets/Desserts: candy, ice cream, frozen yogurt, cake, pastries, doughnuts, cookies, pie, popsicles, jelly, etc.
- Sweet Drinks: soda, punch, lemonade, juice (even 100% juice, even fresh-squeezed), sweet tea, flavored milk, aguas frescas, etc.
- Foods naturally high in sugar: dried fruit (dried cranberries, raisins, dates, etc.), fruit smoothies, etc.
- Sauces made with a lot of sugar: ketchup, BBQ sauce, teriyaki sauce, etc.

Artificial Sweeteners

This is a controversial topic, however, I believe eating food as close to what our ancestors ate is *always* safest. Artificial sweeteners rely on chemicals that trick our body into tasting sweet. The more sweet you taste, the more your taste buds prefer sweet.

"Artificial sweeteners, precisely because they are sweet, encourage sugar craving and sugar dependence. Repeated exposure trains flavor preference. A strong correlation exists between a person's customary intake of a flavor and his preferred intensity for that flavor."[8]

The less we expose ourselves to sweet tastes, from naturally sweet foods or artificial sweeteners, the less our taste buds will crave them.

For many years it was believed that artificial sweeteners do not *and cannot* raise the blood sugar. But a recent study has flipped this thinking upside down when it was revealed that people who consume the most artificial sweeteners were more likely to have blood sugar problems. It appears that artificial sweeteners interact with the microbes in our gut (probiotics), which leads to elevations in blood sugar. In one study, people saw a two-to four-fold increase in blood sugar after consuming artificial sweeteners (aspartame, sucralose, and saccharin were tested in this particular study).[9]

Artificial sweeteners don't just change the bacteria in our gut, they can actually kill them. This is particularly true for Splenda (sucralose), which after only 12 weeks of use has been shown to significantly decrease populations of total anaerobes, bifidobacteria, lactobacilli, *Bacteroides*, clostridia, and total aerobic bacteria.[10] This happened with daily doses only one fifth of the "safe" level set by the FDA (called the Acceptable Daily Intake).

There is so little we understand about how microbes affect our body, but it's a growing area of research, especially in the world of prenatal health. I believe it's best to do everything we can to support the natural and healthy populations of bacteria in our body. Probiotics have far reaching effects on immunity, glycemic control, allergies, nutrient absorption, and of course, normal digestion. I explore this topic in more detail in Chapter 6.

I suggest avoiding artificial sweeteners and simply getting used to things tasting less sweet. When you need an occasional treat, eat a small amount of the real thing.

Artificial Sweeteners to Avoid:
- Aspartame
- Sucralose
- Saccharin
- Acesulfame potassium
- Neotame

Safe Alternatives to Artificial Sweeteners:
Stevia is a safer option to consider as a sugar replacement, since this sweetener is derived from an herb, not a chemistry lab. Stevia-derived sweeteners are generally considered safe during pregnancy.

Small quantities of sugar alcohols are likely also safe, particularly xylitol and erythritol, although like anything sweet, it's best to minimize consumption. Some sugar alcohols can lead to digestive discomfort, such as gas and bloating, so don't go overboard!

Trans Fats

Trans fats are created when food companies take liquid vegetable oil and convert it into a solid when making shortening and margarine. They are the result of a process called "partial hydrogenation" and they show up in processed and fried foods because they extend shelf life and last for a long time (so fast food joints don't have to replace the frying oil as often and Twinkies never go bad).

Unfortunately, these "partially hydrogenated oils" are quite harmful to our health. Not only are they linked to diabetes and cardiovascular disease outside of pregnancy, but they are known to contribute to adverse pregnancy outcomes. Trans fats worsen insulin resistance, meaning your body has more trouble bringing your blood sugar down. Their consumption during pregnancy is linked to asthma and vision problems in infants. They have also been linked to fetal loss by interfering with normal placental function.[11]

Be vigilant about trans fats. Avoid foods made with partially hydrogenated oils such as shortening, margarine, fried foods, fast food, doughnuts, cakes, cookies, and pastries. You'll need to read the ingredients to ensure there are no hidden partially hydrogenated oils, because a labeling loophole allows food companies to include less than half a gram of trans fats *per serving* in products and still list (and advertise) "zero grams trans fats" or "trans fat free" on the packaging.

PECAN SHORTBREAD
COOKIES *trans fat*

Ingredients: Enriched Wheat Flour (Wheat Flour, Niacin, Reduced Iron, Thiamine Mononitrate, Riboflavin, Folic Acid), Partially Hydrogenated Soybean Oil with Citric Acid added as a preservative, Sugar, Egg Whites, Pecans, Baking Soda, Dextrose Monohydrate, Cornstarch, Soy Lecithin, Salt, Natural & Artificial Vanilla Flavor (Water, Ethyl Alcohol, Corn Syrup, Caramel Color, Propylene Glycol), Natural & Artificial Butter Flavor (Corn Oil, Vitamin E), Dried Non Fat Milk.

Summary

If this is all new and overwhelming, don't worry. What seems challenging today will become second nature a few weeks from now. Start by looking at how many carbohydrates you eat in a day. Then apply The Plate Method to your meals and notice how your body feels and how your blood sugar responds. Become mindful of your hunger and fullness cues. Make it a priority to include more real food in your diet and minimize your intake of processed and sugary foods.

This is your chance to get really curious about how food affects your body and to play around with what works and what doesn't. This is a process of self-discovery. Think of it like an experiment rather than a final exam. You'll be learning as you go, taking notes, and adjusting day to day. Don't be upset if you have some high blood sugar numbers during the first few weeks. That's inevitable. At the same time, you'll find meals that result in perfectly normal blood sugar! When you learn what *doesn't* work for you, you learn what *does*.

In the next chapter, we'll discuss how all of these foods fit within a well-balanced meal plan for gestational diabetes.

Chapter 4

Design Your Perfect Meal Plan

By now you've started monitoring your blood sugar and perhaps you've changed the way you're eating. You've probably noticed certain foods make your blood sugar go high and others that keep your blood sugar on an even keel.

That's fantastic because the key to successfully navigating a pregnancy complicated with gestational diabetes is paying attention to your blood sugar and knowing how food sustains, raises, or lowers it. Everybody's blood sugar response is unique, but as you learned in the last chapter, some general guidelines hold true.

In this chapter, I'll give you three sample meal plans with differing levels of carbohydrates. The meal plan you choose will depend on your blood sugar, how many carbohydrates your body is used to eating, and if you need to gain or maintain your weight at this stage in your pregnancy.

If your body is accustomed to a very-low-carbohydrate diet, such as a low-carb Paleo or ketogenic style diet, I suggest the lower range of carbohydrates. If all of this carbohydrate talk is completely new to you or you've never considered monitoring the amount of carbohydrates in your diet, I suggest choosing the highest carbohydrate plan I provide and then modifying as needed for your blood sugar control.

Our goals for this plan are not only to keep your blood sugar in the normal range, but to also provide enough essential vitamins, minerals, and other nutrients for your developing baby (more on those special foods/nutrients in Chapter 5). These are general guidelines and you are encouraged to work with your healthcare practitioner to customize a plan for you. Your perfect diet might be higher or lower in carbohydrates than the ones I present here. For years, I was taught that women needed a minimum of 175g of carbohydrates per day in the second and third trimester of pregnancy, but I've come to understand that this recommendation lacks evidence and efficacy in clinical practice. The old argument that you need a high carbohydrate diet to avoid going into "ketosis" or spilling ketones in your urine is outdated and I explore more on this subject in Chapter 11 if you're interested in the research.

Individualization is paramount, but in general, a lower amount of carbohydrates is needed to achieve normal blood sugar without necessitating the use of insulin or medication. That said, some women can handle higher amounts of carbohydrates without experiencing high blood sugar. If that's you and you feel energized, satisfied, and are gaining weight normally (and your baby is growing normally), then by all means, continue on that diet.

However, if your blood sugar levels are high enough that your healthcare provider is suggesting you start insulin or medication, adjusting your diet to be lower in carbohydrates is a safe and practical first step to revealing if you can do this with diet (and exercise) alone.

If you are already on insulin and medication, you should consult your healthcare provider before significantly decreasing the amount of carbohydrates you eat, as these medicines, by design, lower your blood sugar. Without eating the same level of carbohydrates consistently while on these medicines, you risk your blood sugar going too low, which is a risk to you and your baby. If you *do* decide to reduce your carbohydrates, do so *gradually* and with the knowledge that your medication dosages and timing may need to be adjusted.

Believe me, I don't expect you to follow any of the meal plans to the "T." These are merely a way to apply the nutrition principles described previously into a well-balanced, real food meal plan. You're encouraged to get creative in the kitchen and get comfortable with cooking low-carbohydrate, nutrient-dense meals.

Real Food Meal Plans

The following real food meal plans show you how you can modify your diet to be higher or lower in carbohydrates. The foods marked in bold indicate either an additional food or simply an adjustment in the portion size to increase the carbohydrate level among the 90g, 120g, and 150g of carbohydrate meal plans. You might be surprised at how easy it is to accidentally eat a high-carbohydrate diet when you thought you were eating low carb.

Some of the dishes listed have an accompanying recipe in Appendix A. For additional GD-friendly recipes and meal ideas, visit **www.RealFoodforGD.com**.

SAMPLE MEAL PLAN - DAY 1

Meal	90g Carbs	120g Carbs	150g Carbs
Breakfast	1 cup Greek yogurt (full-fat, unsweetened) 1/2 cup blueberries 1/4 cup macadamia nuts Stevia (optional, to taste) Vanilla extract (to taste) (16g net carbs)	1 cup Greek yogurt (full-fat, unsweetened) 1/2 cup blueberries 1/4 cup macadamia nuts Stevia (optional, to taste) Vanilla extract (to taste) (16g net carbs)	1 cup Greek yogurt (full-fat, unsweetened) **3/4 cup blueberries** 1/4 cup macadamia nuts Stevia (optional, to taste) Vanilla extract (to taste) (20g net carbs)
Lunch	1 cup beanless beef chili Sour cream Salsa Green onions 1/2 avocado Fresh lime (14g net carbs)	1 cup beanless beef chili Sour cream Salsa Green onions 1/2 avocado Fresh lime (14g net carbs)	1 cup beanless beef chili **1/2 cup pinto beans** Sour cream Salsa Green onions 1/2 avocado Fresh lime (29g net carbs)
Dinner	3oz salmon salad in romaine lettuce wraps Sliced cucumber and carrot Side salad + dressing Small handful sliced almonds (18g net carbs)	3oz salmon salad in romaine lettuce wraps Sliced cucumber and carrot Side salad + dressing Small handful sliced almonds **1/2 cup fresh pineapple** (28g net carbs)	3oz salmon salad in romaine lettuce wraps Sliced cucumber and carrot Side salad + dressing Small handful sliced almonds **1/2 cup fresh pineapple** (28g net carbs)
Snacks	Olives + cherry tomatoes + mozzarella cheese Guacamole + sliced veggies Hard boiled egg (0-10g net carbs each)	Olives + cherry tomatoes + mozzarella cheese Guacamole + sliced veggies + **1 oz organic corn chips** Hard boiled egg + **1 slice sprouted grain bread** + butter (5-18g net carbs each)	Olives + cherry tomatoes + mozzarella cheese Guacamole + sliced veggies + **1 oz organic corn chips** Hard boiled egg + **1 slice sprouted grain bread +** butter (5-18g net carbs each)
Dessert (optional)	Homemade berry sorbet (10g net carbs)	Homemade berry sorbet (10g net carbs)	Homemade berry sorbet (10g net carbs)

SAMPLE MEAL PLAN - DAY 2

Meal	90g Carbs	120g Carbs	150g Carbs
Breakfast	2 eggs 1-2 Tbsp butter 1 cup sauteed kale 1/2 cup sliced tomatoes (8g net carbs)	2 eggs 1-2 Tbsp butter 1 cup sauteed kale 1/2 cup sliced tomatoes **1 slice sprouted grain toast or 1/2 cup cooked sweet potato** (23g net carbs)	2 eggs 1-2 Tbsp butter 1 cup sauteed kale 1/2 cup sliced tomatoes **1 slice sprouted grain toast or 1/2 cup cooked sweet potato** (23g net carbs)
Lunch	Green salad (3+ cups) 2 Tbsp oil & vinegar dressing 1/2 avocado 1/2 cup sliced vegetables 3 oz chicken or salmon 1/2 cup blueberries (25g net carbs)	Green salad (3+ cups) 2 Tbsp oil & vinegar dressing 1/2 avocado 1/2 cup sliced vegetables 3 oz chicken or salmon **1/2 cup roasted beets** 1/2 cup blueberries (31g net carbs)	Green salad (3+ cups) 2 Tbsp oil & vinegar dressing 1/2 avocado 1/2 cup sliced vegetables 3 oz chicken or salmon **1/2 cup roasted beets 1/2 cup butternut squash** 1/2 cup blueberries (43g net carbs)
Dinner	3-4 oz Slow-cooker carnitas Tomato salsa Sour cream Riced cauliflower Roasted bell peppers and onions (18g net carbs)	3-4 oz Slow-cooker carnitas Tomato salsa Sour cream Riced cauliflower **1/2 cup black beans** Roasted bell peppers and onions (33g net carbs)	3-4 oz Slow-cooker carnitas Tomato salsa Sour cream Riced cauliflower **3/4 cup black beans** Roasted bell peppers and onions (38g net carbs)
Snacks	Small handful of almonds + 1/2 peach or nectarine 2 oz cheese 1/2 cup plain greek yogurt + vanilla extract + stevia (optional) + 1/2 cup strawberries (0-15g net carbs each)	Small handful of almonds + **1 peach or nectarine** 2 oz cheese + **6 whole grain crackers** 1/2 cup plain greek yogurt + vanilla extract + stevia (optional) + 1/2 cup strawberries (8-20g net carbs)	Small handful of almonds + **1 peach or nectarine** 2 oz cheese + **6-10 whole grain crackers** 1/2 cup plain greek yogurt + vanilla extract + stevia (optional) + 1/2 cup strawberries + **1 tsp honey** (12-22g net carbs)
Dessert (optional)	1 oz dark chocolate (75% cocoa or more) (5g net carbs)	1 oz dark chocolate (75% cocoa or more) (5g net carbs)	1 oz dark chocolate (75% cocoa or more) (5g net carbs)

SAMPLE MEAL PLAN - DAY 3

Meal	90g Carbs	120g Carbs	150g Carbs
Breakfast	Crustless spinach quiche 1-2 breakfast sausages Grated parmesan cheese 1/3 medium banana (12g net carbs)	Crustless spinach quiche 1-2 breakfast sausages Grated parmesan cheese **1/2 medium banana** (17g net carbs)	Crustless spinach quiche 1-2 breakfast sausages Grated parmesan cheese **1/2 medium banana** (17g net carbs)
Lunch	2 cups homemade chicken + vegetable soup Side salad Shredded cheese (20g net carbs)	2 cups homemade chicken + vegetable soup **1/2 cup cooked lentils** (mixed into soup) Side salad Shredded cheese (32g net carbs)	2 cups homemade chicken + vegetable soup **3/4 cup cooked lentils** (mixed into soup) Side salad Shredded cheese (40g net carbs)
Dinner	3-4oz grass-fed beef meatloaf Roasted celery, carrots, & onions 1/2 cup sautéed spinach 1 Tbsp butter (22g net carbs)	3-4oz grass-fed beef meatloaf Roasted celery, carrots, & onions 1/2 cup sautéed spinach 1 Tbsp butter **1/2 cup sweet potato fries** (36g net carbs)	3-4oz grass-fed beef meatloaf Roasted celery, carrots, & onions 1/2 cup sautéed spinach 1 Tbsp butter **1/2 cup sweet potato fries** **1 Tbsp ketchup** (41g net carbs)
Snacks	Celery, cucumber, zucchini + 1/2 cup hummus 1 small apple + nut butter Beef or turkey jerky (5-16g net carbs each)	Celery, cucumber, zucchini, **carrots** + 1/2 cup hummus 1 **medium** apple + nut butter Beef or turkey jerky (5-20g net carbs)	Celery, cucumber, zucchini, **carrots** + 1/2 cup hummus 1 **medium** apple + nut butter Beef or turkey jerky (5-20g net carbs)
Dessert (optional)	1/2 cup raspberries + homemade whipped cream (sweetened with stevia) (5g net carbs)	1/2 cup raspberries + **1/2** **fresh peach** + homemade whipped cream (sweetened with stevia) (14g net carbs)	1/2 cup raspberries + **1/2** **fresh peach** + homemade whipped cream (sweetened with stevia) (14g net carbs)

SAMPLE MEAL PLAN - DAY 4

Meal	90g Carbs	120g Carbs	150g Carbs
Breakfast	1 cup full-fat cottage cheese 1/2 cup chopped fresh fruit Small handful pecans Dash of cinnamon Stevia (optional, to taste) (18g net carbs)	1 cup full-fat cottage cheese 1/2 cup chopped fresh fruit Small handful pecans Dash of cinnamon Stevia (optional, to taste) (18g net carbs)	1 cup full-fat cottage cheese 1/2 cup chopped fresh fruit Small handful pecans Dash of cinnamon Stevia (optional, to taste) (18g net carbs)
Lunch	1 cup spaghetti squash 1/2 cup tomato-cream sauce 3 grassfed beef meatballs 1/2 cup cooked broccoli Fresh basil Parmesan cheese (28g net carbs)	1 cup spaghetti squash 1/2 cup tomato-cream sauce 3 grassfed beef meatballs 1/2 cup cooked broccoli Fresh basil Parmesan cheese **1 slice whole grain garlic bread** (43g net carbs)	1 cup spaghetti squash 1/2 cup tomato-cream sauce 3 grassfed beef meatballs 1/2 cup cooked broccoli Fresh basil Parmesan cheese **1 slice whole grain garlic bread** (43g net carbs)
Dinner	4oz coconut chicken curry 1/2 cup roasted curried cauliflower 1/2 cup sauteed spinach 1 Tbsp butter (25g net carbs)	4oz coconut chicken curry 1/2 cup roasted curried cauliflower 1/2 cup sauteed spinach 1 Tbsp butter **1/2 cup cooked potatoes** (40g net carbs)	4oz coconut chicken curry 1/2 cup roasted curried cauliflower 1/2 cup sauteed spinach 1 Tbsp butter **1/2 cup cooked potatoes** (40g net carbs)
Snacks	Sliced bell peppers, snap peas + 1/4 cup sour cream dip Sardines packed in olive oil + celery Nutty "Granola" Bar (5-16g net carbs each)	Sliced bell peppers, snap peas + 1/4 cup sour cream dip Sardines packed in olive oil + **6 brown rice crackers** Nutty "Granola" Bar (5-16g net carbs each)	Sliced bell peppers, snap peas + 1/4 cup sour cream dip Sardines packed in olive oil + **6 brown rice crackers** Nutty "Granola" Bar (5-16g net carbs each)
Dessert (optional)	1 dark chocolate peanut butter cup (9g net carbs)	1 dark chocolate peanut butter cup (9g net carbs)	1 dark chocolate peanut butter cup (9g net carbs)

47

SAMPLE MEAL PLAN – DAY 5

Meal	90g Carbs	120g Carbs	150g Carbs
Breakfast	3/4 cup grain-free granola 1 cup unsweetened almond milk	3/4 cup grain-free granola 1 cup unsweetened almond milk	3/4 cup grain-free granola 1 cup unsweetened almond milk **1/2 cup strawberries**
	(14g net carbs)	(14g net carbs)	(19g net carbs)
Lunch	Caprese salad: 2 cups fresh spinach, sliced mozzarella, tomatoes, cucumber, basil 2 Tbsp olive oil + balsamic vinegar dressing	Caprese salad: 2 cups fresh spinach, sliced mozzarella, tomatoes, cucumber, basil 2 Tbsp olive oil + balsamic vinegar dressing **1/2 cup homemade croutons (use wholegrain bread)**	Caprese salad: 2 cups fresh spinach, sliced mozzarella, tomatoes, cucumber, basil 2 Tbsp olive oil + balsamic vinegar dressing **3/4 cup homemade croutons (use wholegrain bread)**
	(24g net carbs)	(36g net carbs)	(42g net carbs)
Dinner	4oz low-carb shepherd's pie 1/2 cup roasted broccoli 1 Tbsp butter	4oz low-carb shepherd's pie 1/2 cup roasted broccoli 1 Tbsp butter **1/2 cup mashed sweet potatoes**	4oz low-carb shepherd's pie 1/2 cup roasted broccoli 1 Tbsp butter **1/2 cup mashed sweet potatoes**
	(25g net carbs)	40g net carbs)	(40g net carbs)
Snacks	Small handful cashews + 1/2 cup blackberries	Small handful cashews + 1/2 cup blackberries	Small handful cashews + 1/2 cup blackberries
	Celery + organic peanut butter	Celery + organic peanut butter	Celery + organic peanut butter
	1/2 cup sweet potato fries + 1 oz grilled chicken	1/2 cup sweet potato fries + 1 oz grilled chicken	1/2 cup sweet potato fries + 1 oz grilled chicken
	(5-16g net carbs each)	(5-16g net carbs each)	(5-16g net carbs each)
Dessert (optional)	2 coconut macaroons	2 coconut macaroons	2 coconut macaroons
	(15g net carbs)	(15g net carbs)	(15g net carbs)

48

Breakfast

You'll notice all of the breakfast options are lower in carbohydrates than lunch or dinner. That's because most women experience more insulin resistance in the morning, partly due to a surge in placental hormones and cortisol early in the day. So if you eat a high-carbohydrate breakfast, sometimes your body can have trouble bringing your blood sugar down to normal. (So long, waffles and cereal!) I suggest trying a breakfast with approximately 15 grams of carbohydrates until you know how your body responds.

Also, some women are more sensitive to the carbohydrates in fruit (fructose) and milk (lactose) in the morning, so you may need to omit one or both of these foods from breakfast. In general, lower sugar fruits, like berries, are well tolerated. Similarly, low-lactose dairy products, such as Greek yogurt, cheese, cottage cheese, butter, and heavy cream are rarely an issue (but milk and regular yogurt can be problematic).

Lunch and Dinner

At lunch and dinner, I suggest applying The Plate Method as outlined in the previous chapter. Vegetables are *always* included at lunch and dinner and should make up the majority of your plate. A source of protein and fat should also be included with each meal. Your carbohydrate tolerance will vary. Some women can only eat 15 grams of carbohydrates without experiencing high blood sugar, while others can eat as much as 45 grams without a problem. If your blood sugar is coming out high after lunch or dinner, I suggest you reduce your portions of high-carbohydrate foods (grains/starches, fruit, and milk) and instead aim for most of your carbohydrates to come from non-starchy vegetables. There are more tips and tricks to fine-tuning your plan in Chapter 9.

Snacks

With gestational diabetes, it's important to keep your portions at meals in check so you don't have high blood sugar after eating. This usually means you'll be hungry for a snack between meals. Having a variety of healthy snacks to choose from will keep your blood sugar and your taste buds happy.

Snacks can help you eat slightly less at meals (preventing a spike in blood sugar), and also prevent you from getting too hungry (preventing low blood sugar between meals).

Be sure your snacks *always* contain a source of protein and fat, so they keep you satisfied. Eating *just* carbohydrates for a snack, such as crackers or a piece of fruit ("naked carbohydrates"), tends to cause a spike followed by a steep drop in blood sugar, making you even *more* hungry by the time you're ready for your next meal. So, instead of plain crackers, match them with some cheese. And instead of a lone apple, pair it with some peanut butter.

In general, plan to have 3 snacks per day, 1) between breakfast and lunch, 2) between lunch and dinner, and 3) after dinner (bedtime). The bedtime snack is critical because this may help lower your fasting blood sugar the following morning. If you have high fasting blood sugar, be sure to read Chapter 9.

Low Carb Snack Ideas: (barely raise the blood sugar, if at all)

- Nuts - any kind (almonds, cashews, walnuts, pecans, etc.)
- ½ cup plain Greek yogurt + ¼ cup berries (may use stevia to sweeten)
- Beef or turkey jerky (look for one without MSG)
- Cheddar, jack, or string cheese
- ¼ cup blueberries or strawberries with unsweetened whipped cream
- Guacamole + fresh celery and bell pepper
- Small salad with pine nuts, balsamic dressing, and goat cheese
- Hard boiled egg + salt and pepper
- Cherry tomatoes, mozzarella, fresh basil, olive oil + vinegar
- Olives and dill pickles
- Kale chips + nuts
- ½ avocado with salt, pepper, and lemon juice
- Grilled chicken breast with pesto and Parmesan cheese
- Sardines + cucumber and bell pepper slices
- Roasted curried cauliflower with coconut milk + cashews
- Celery sticks with peanut butter or almond butter
- 1 oz dark chocolate + nuts (75% cacao or more. The darker, the better!)
- Grass-fed beef patty with cheese served over a green salad
- Sautéed kale with real bacon
- ¼ cup raspberries + ricotta or cottage cheese (stevia to sweeten)
- Dry salami + cheddar cheese + cherry tomatoes

Moderate Carb Snack Ideas: (raise the blood sugar a little)

- ½ cup homemade sweet potato fries + grilled chicken
- Quesadilla – 1 small corn tortilla + cheese + avocado + salsa/cilantro, full-fat sour cream
- Taco – 1 small corn tortilla + chicken, beef, fish, or shrimp + lettuce/cabbage, salsa, full-fat sour cream
- ½ cup beans or lentils + cheese
- Whole grain crackers + cheese or peanut butter
- Whole grain crackers + sardines
- Medium apple + small handful of almonds or string cheese
- ½ banana + peanut butter
- ½ cup fresh pineapple + cottage cheese
- ½ cup fruited/flavored Greek yogurt
- 1 cup milk + small handful of almonds
- ½ cup hummus + feta cheese (pasteurized) + celery/carrot sticks
- ½ peanut butter sandwich on sprouted whole grain bread
- ½ sandwich with turkey or cheese (+ mustard, lettuce, tomato…)
- Smoothie: ¼ c berries, ½ c plain Greek yogurt, 1 cup unsweetened almond milk. Stevia or vanilla extract to taste. (bonus points for adding 1 Tbsp chia seeds!)

Drinks

Let's face it, drinking *just* water can get old. So here are some things to keep in mind when you're planning what to drink.

Many drinks are a hidden source of carbohydrates. Take juice, for example. An 8 ounce glass of juice has around 30g of carbohydrates, even the freshly squeezed, raw, with-the-pulp organic kind! That amount of sugar is equivalent to what's in 8 ounces of soda. Even though the source is natural and fresh juice comes with more nutrients than soda, your blood sugar will respond almost identically. You'll still see your blood sugar sky-rocket!

My suggestion with drinks is to avoid *any* with naturally occurring or added sugars, so you have more room in your diet to *eat* your carbohydrates. Below are some examples of acceptable beverages. These are all low in carbohydrates with the exception of dairy milk.

- Unsweetened almond or coconut milk
- Whole milk (each 8 oz glass contains 12g carbs)
- Infused water: a great way to add flavor without too much sugar
    - cucumber + lime
    - grapefruit + blueberries
    - peach + basil
    - strawberries or blackberries
    - orange, lemon, lime
    - strawberry + kiwi
    - apple + cinnamon sticks
    - mint + lime
    - pear + fresh ginger slices
- Sparkling water (flavored is ok, but make sure it's unsweetened)
- Up to 3 cups of unsweetened black, green, or white tea (or 6-12oz coffee)*
- Mint, ginger, or raspberry leaf tea
- Hot chocolate (made with unsweetened almond milk, unsweetened cocoa powder, and stevia)

* Caffeinated drinks are best limited. Generally, it's suggested pregnant women not exceed 200mg of caffeine per day.

Summary

Now that you have some ideas for meals, snacks, and beverages, it's time to create your perfect meal plan. Feel free to mix and match meals from different days. Let your feelings of hunger guide when and how much you eat; just pay attention to your blood sugar, so you can adjust your meal plan as needed.

Of course, there are important nutrients to think about beyond carbohydrates. In the next chapter, I'll be discussing the foods to emphasize during pregnancy that play a special role in fetal development and help keep this pregnancy as low risk as possible.

Chapter 5

Special Foods and Nutrients for Pregnancy

Real Foods to Emphasize During Pregnancy

Many women intuitively feel that they should be eating certain foods to nourish their growing baby. Indeed, traditional cultures from around the globe each had unique foods that were prized before, during, and after pregnancy. In our modern culture, we've lost the connection with these traditions and focus instead on individual nutrients. But focusing on one little piece rather than the whole food from which it is sourced ignores many other nutrients, known and unknown, something that's been referred to as "nutritionism."

So in this chapter, we will focus primarily on the *food*. The foods I review in this chapter have hundreds of years of use in our diets. Modern science is just beginning to reveal *why* these foods serve such an important role in our health. I will point out which nutrients are abundant in these foods and how they support fetal development.

You may wonder why this chapter comes after the nutrition and meal planning chapters. The reason is simple. Focusing first on awareness of which foods contain carbohydrates and how to fit that into a palatable, well-balanced meal plan that normalizes your blood sugar is priority number one. Then ensuring that these foods are nutrient-dense is priority number two. Too often, we can become distracted by the promise of certain foods being a "magic bullet," but there is no such thing, so we need to start with the basics (limiting carbohydrates) and add on nutrient-dense foods from there.

Ideally, with this information you'll be able to consciously and intelligently modify your meals to meet all of your nutrient needs *and* satisfy your taste buds. After all, enjoying what we're eating is part of nourishing ourselves.

Eggs

Eggs are an incredible superfood, especially during pregnancy. Not only are they a convenient source of protein, but they are excellent sources of many vitamins and minerals commonly lacking in a prenatal diet. Eggs from chickens raised on pasture (meaning outdoors, in grass, pecking at insects and enjoying the sunlight) are much more nutrient-dense than conventionally-produced eggs.

Here are a few ways eggs from pastured chickens are superior:[12]
- Vitamin A content is 30% higher, which is clearly visible from the rich, orange color of the yolks. The more fresh greens, grasses, and bugs a chicken eats, the higher the vitamin A levels
- Vitamin E content is fully double that from commercially-raised hens
- Omega-3 content is 2.5 times higher than eggs from commercially-raised hens. Eggs are one of the few non-seafood sources of DHA, a key omega-3 fat that is linked to higher IQ in infants
- Omega-6 fats are found in lower levels, which is favorable, since these fats tend to cause inflammation (Eggs from pastured chickens have less than half the ratio of omega-6 to omega-3 fatty acids)
- Vitamin D content is 3-6 times higher due to regular sun exposure

I should mention that all of the nutrients discussed above are found in the egg yolk, so do eat the *whole* egg, otherwise you miss out on the benefits. There's a reason an egg comes with a yolk!

Regardless of how the chickens are raised, egg yolks are a rich source of a special nutrient called choline. Choline is a relative of the B-vitamins that hadn't gained much attention until the last 15 years. In fact, the first recommended daily intakes for choline were issued in 1998. It turns out choline has some of the same beneficial effects on a developing baby as folate (also called folic acid in supplements), including fostering normal brain development and preventing neural tube defects.[13] Choline can also permanently change, in a good way, the genetic expression of your growing baby.[14]

"When rat pups receive choline supplements (*in utero* or during the second week of life), their brain function is changed, resulting in lifelong memory enhancement. This change in memory function appears to be due to changes in the development of the memory center (hippocampus) in the brain. These changes are so important that investigators can pick out the groups of animals whose mothers had extra choline even when these animals are elderly. Thus, memory function in the aged is, in part, determined by what mother ate."[15]

Unfortunately, most women only consume a fraction of the recommended daily allowance of choline, partly because food sources are limited or perhaps because they've been scared away from eating egg yolks.[16]

Egg yolks and liver have, by far, the highest concentration of choline compared to any other food. Just two eggs (with the yolks!) per day meets about half of a pregnant woman's needs for choline. That's why eggs are frequently included in the sample meal plans in this book. Egg yolks, by the way, are also a rich source of folate, B-vitamins, antioxidants (including lutein and zeaxanthin, which are crucial to eye and vision development), and many minerals. Choline works synergistically with the omega-3, DHA, enhancing how much DHA is incorporated into cells.[17] It's no accident that eggs are rich in both nutrients.

When you analyze macronutrients, eggs contain only fat and protein (no carbohydrates), so they don't raise the blood sugar. This makes eggs a perfect breakfast option when you have gestational diabetes. If before becoming pregnant, you struggled to maintain your weight or had food cravings during the day, eggs make a wise choice in the morning.

Researchers investigating people's responses to different types of breakfast found that, compared to a bagel, those who ate eggs naturally ate less throughout the day, had fewer cravings, and experienced fewer spikes in blood sugar and insulin.[18] Eggs are full of nutrients, they keep you satisfied, and they stabilize your energy levels. They are a win-win-win.

If you're nervous to eat eggs because you are worried about cholesterol, know that recent research disproved the theory that dietary cholesterol increases the risk of heart disease.[19] And often, the opposite is true! It turns out that excessive dietary carbohydrates are more closely linked to dyslipidemia than dietary cholesterol (or saturated fat).[20] Besides, our brains *need* cholesterol. In fact, 25% of the cholesterol in our bodies is found in the brain where it plays a crucial role in normal neural function. If you want to provide the raw materials to help your baby develop a healthy brain, you should absolutely be consuming cholesterol!

Some women are nervous to consume eggs because they've been told they can cause food poisoning. Food safety concerns over eggs have been overstated again and again, especially to pregnant women. According to the Centers for Disease Control, food poisoning due to eggs accounts for only 2% of all reports nationwide, while plant foods are the cause of 42% of food poisoning cases, with fruit and leafy vegetables cited as the most common culprits.[21] Yet, you never hear health officials warning pregnant moms to avoid fresh fruits and vegetables! Sourcing your eggs from pasture-raised chickens is one of the best ways to reduce the risk of food poisoning, since organic farms have a seven-fold lower rate of *Salmonella* infection compared to commercial producers.[22] Often you can find pastured eggs from local farmers or health food stores.

Liver

Aside from eggs, liver is the only other major dietary source of choline. It also happens to be rich in almost every other vitamin and mineral that modern nutrition science has identified so far. Liver contains iron in a highly-absorbable form, a mineral that most pregnant women need more of to prevent maternal anemia, miscarriage, and premature delivery. Liver is also one of the richest food sources of folate and vitamin B12, both key to maintaining healthy red blood cells and fostering healthy brain development in your baby. Inadequate maternal vitamin B12 has been linked to neural tube defects, spontaneous abortion, and preterm delivery.[23]

Folate is another B vitamin found in liver that's best known for its role in preventing birth defects. Most women seek this vitamin from supplements, but few know that the folate obtained from food is far superior. Due to genetic variations, some women are unable to use the synthetic form of folate, known as folic acid, found in supplements. Eating liver ensures you obtain the form of folate that your body can fully utilize, no matter your genetics. I explore the topic of supplements in greater detail in Chapter 6. Liver is also incredibly rich in fat-soluble vitamins, including vitamins A, D, E, and K; all nutrients that are difficult to obtain otherwise.

Many of you reading this may have been warned not to consume liver during pregnancy, since it is rich in vitamin A. This has sparked controversy over the years, mostly because an old study linked high-dose *synthetic* supplemental vitamin A to birth defects. However, we now know that naturally occurring vitamin A does *not* exert this toxicity, particularly when consumed with adequate vitamin D and vitamin K2, nutrients that are also found in abundance in liver.[24] This illustrates perfectly why obtaining nutrients from food is far safer than getting them from supplements.

"Liver and supplements are *not* of equivalent teratogenic potential [risk of causing birth defects]. Advice to pregnant women on the consumption of liver based on the reported teratogenicity of vitamin A supplements should be reconsidered."[25]

Ongoing concerns over vitamin A toxicity are perplexing considering deficiency is fairly common in pregnant women.

One screening study found that fully one third of pregnant women were borderline deficient, despite having access to plenty of vitamin A-rich foods.[26] This essential nutrient is widely recognized for its role in normal growth and development during pregnancy, including the developing lungs, kidneys, heart, eyes, and other organs. Even the National Institutes of Health states "Pregnant women need extra vitamin A for fetal growth and tissue maintenance and for supporting their own metabolism." Certainly, excessive amounts of any nutrient is problematic, and vitamin A being fat soluble does raise the risk of toxicity, but that does not defend the recommendation to avoid our most valuable food source of the vitamin.

"Pregnant women or those considering becoming pregnant are generally advised to avoid the intake of vitamin-A rich liver and liver foods, based upon unsupported scientific findings."[26]

I should also mention that plant sources of vitamin A are not equivalent to animal sources. Plant sources, such as sweet potato, carrots, and kale contain carotenoids (provitamin A) and although our bodies theoretically can convert provitamin A into true vitamin A (retinol), the conversion rate is highly variable person to person, partly influenced by genetics.[27]

"A summary of the major human studies that determined conversion factors for dietary β-carotene to retinol … show that the conversion efficiency of dietary β-carotene to retinol is in the range of 3.6–28:1 by weight. There is a wide variation in conversion factors reported not only between different studies but also between individuals in a particular study."[28]

And paradoxically, the more beta-carotene you eat, the *less* you convert to vitamin A.[29] That means you indeed need *some* dietary sources of preformed vitamin A to ensure enough for yourself and your growing baby. Consuming a few ounces of liver once or twice a week is sufficient along with the carotenes from vegetables, and the other dietary sources of vitamin A (grass-fed butter, animal fats from pasture-raised animals, egg yolks, etc.). Unless we're talking polar bear liver, which is unique in that it *does* have excessive amounts of vitamin A, the benefits outweigh the risks when it comes to eating liver. Just remember to source it from healthy, pasture-raised animals.

If you're not used to eating liver or dislike the taste, be sure to read through the recipes in Appendix A. It can easily be "hidden" in recipes, such as meatloaf, meatballs, or shepherd's pie.

Bone Broth, Meat on the Bone, and Slow-Cooked Meat

Chances are your grandmother knew how to make soup from scratch, but now most of us grab a can or carton of "broth" at the store instead. Homemade broths made from bones are not just a way to save money on food, but a valuable source of nutrients otherwise lacking in our diets. Traditional cultures didn't eat boneless, skinless chicken breasts and throw out the rest of the animal. They ate the organs, the fat, and they used any tough cuts of meat, bones and skin to make soup.

Once again, modern research is showing us that this practice is something we should return to. The bones, skin, and connective tissues of animals are rich in protein, gelatin, collagen, glycine, and minerals. Bones contain more minerals per ounce than any other body tissue, and long, slow simmering helps to leach those minerals into the broth. That makes bone broth a great source of calcium, magnesium, iron, zinc, potassium, and many trace minerals. By the way, if you're not much of a meat eater, bone broth is a great way to get protein and iron!

Let's explore some of the other benefits of broth and slow-cooked meats. The gelatin and collagen in these foods are rich in an important amino acid called glycine. Glycine is generally not discussed because it's "conditionally essential," meaning the body can make plenty from other amino acids. However, pregnancy is a special case where the body may require additional glycine from the diet. Researchers have found that "the demand for glycine during pregnancy may already exceed the capacity for its synthesis, making it conditionally indispensable."[30] Glycine needs tend to increase as pregnancy progresses and this amino acid is needed for the synthesis of fetal DNA and collagen, among other functions.

"As pregnancy advances, the endogenous production of glycine may be insufficient to satisfy the increasing demands."[31]

Glycine, however, is not abundant in lean meats, skinless poultry, dairy products, or vegetarian sources of protein. Moreover, eating exclusively from the above foods for your protein needs may provide excessive methionine, an amino acid that reduces glycine stores and may be toxic in large quantities.[30] Excess methionine has been linked to high homocysteine, neural tube defects, preeclampsia, spontaneous abortion, and premature delivery.[32]

"Diets with an inappropriate balance of methionine can adversely affect both short-term reproductive function and the long-term physiology of the offspring. The catabolism of unused methionine increases the demand for glycine and may cause a deficiency."[30]

It remains that making bone broth, slow-cooking tough cuts of meat, and leaving the skin on poultry are the best way to ensure you get enough glycine. Gelatin is naturally very rich in glycine, so one option is to add pure gelatin powder to other foods (not the pre-sweetened kind, of course!).

Few studies are done on humans that purposefully restrict intake of essential nutrients during pregnancy for obvious ethical reasons, but these studies are still performed on lab rats. When rats are fed a diet low in protein, their offspring develop cardiovascular problems and high blood pressure. However, when low protein diets are supplemented with glycine, these effects are not seen. Researchers comment, "The availability of glycine appears to be of critical importance for normal cardiovascular development." In addition, "poor glycine status has been suggested in preterm infants."[33]

Inadequate maternal intake of glycine and other sulfur-containing amino acids in humans predisposes their offspring to develop type 2 diabetes and high blood pressure later in life.[34]

Clearly the availability of glycine is of crucial importance. We also know that choline and glycine are related in their functions in the body. Choline may be converted into glycine if the diet is not sufficient. Of course, that assumes a mom is also obtaining enough choline, a nutrient that most women don't even have on their radar.

Another benefit of glycine is that it's required in the production of glutathione, one of the body's most powerful detoxification enzymes which helps to naturally detoxify chemicals we encounter on a daily basis.

Let's not forget that bone broth and slow-cooked meats provide much more than just glycine. The collagen is also important, as the body's need for collagen increases throughout pregnancy. "Quantitative collagen determinations demonstrate an increase of approximately 800 percent in the collagen content of the human uterus at term as compared with the non-pregnant state."[35]

Just like liver, be sure to source your meat and bones from pasture-raised and grass-fed animals whenever possible.

Vegetables, Especially the Leafy Green Kind

This may be the most obvious of the foods to emphasize when you're expecting. Green, leafy vegetables have many advantages, primarily because they are concentrated in vitamins, minerals, and antioxidants while being low in carbohydrates. Researchers have identified 45 different flavonoids (a type of antioxidant) in kale alone.
The folate that you're told to get enough of comes from the word "foliage," meaning leaves. Indeed, leafy greens are one

of the richest sources of dietary folate (as are the meat and eggs of animals that eat plenty of foliage). Greens also contain vitamin C, beta-carotene, fiber, many B-vitamins, and trace minerals. Vitamin C works synergistically with amino acids and other nutrients to maintain normal collagen production.

Greens have high amounts of vitamin K1, which plays a crucial role in normal blood clotting. They are also high in two nutrients that may prevent or ease the severity of morning sickness: vitamin B6 and magnesium. Potassium is also fairly high in greens, a key mineral that helps you maintain normal blood pressure and prevents swelling.

Keep in mind the nutrients in all vegetables, especially the antioxidants and fat-soluble vitamins, are best absorbed when you eat them with some fat, so don't be shy about adding grass-fed butter, coconut oil, olive oil, avocado, nuts, or other fats to your vegetables.[36] Certain nutrients are better absorbed when vegetables are raw, while some are enhanced when the vegetable is cooked. For that reason, I recommend eating a combination of cooked and raw vegetables. Ideally, purchase organically grown vegetables to minimize exposure to pesticide residues.

Salmon, Fatty Fish, and Other Seafood

With increased awareness about mercury and other contaminants in fish, some women have been told not to consume fish while pregnant. Unfortunately this information is a little misguided. There *are* certain fish that are very high in mercury and should be avoided, which includes tuna, swordfish, king mackerel, and shark. Many other types of fish are perfectly safe to eat while pregnant, even if they contain a small amount of mercury, and here's why.

Fish also contains high amounts of selenium, a mineral that readily binds with mercury, thereby preventing it from exerting toxic effects in the body.[37] Still, I recommend becoming aware of the types of fish and seafood that contain high levels of mercury and instead eating the fish with the lowest levels, which are generally smaller fish.[38]

"Mercury levels showed significant positive correlations with fish size for ten species. Size was the best predictor of mercury levels."[38]

Hopefully, this little known fact about selenium will lessen some fears about eating fish, because there are many good reasons to consume it, as I'll review below.

Cold water fish are rich in omega-3s, especially the difficult to obtain form called DHA. This omega-3 fatty acid is crucial for optimal brain and vision development, as I'll explore in more detail in Chapter 6.

Aside from DHA, fatty fish and seafood are also among the few foods rich in vitamin D, a nutrient that most pregnant women are deficient in.[39] Seafood also contains many trace minerals, including iodine and zinc. Iodine needs are increased by 50% during pregnancy and deficiency is common.[40] Iodine is necessary for normal thyroid function in both mother and fetus, and is essential to healthy brain development. According to the *Journal of the American Medical Association*, "Iodine deficiency remains the leading cause of preventable intellectual disability worldwide."[41] Consuming foods from the ocean -- in particular, seaweed, scallops, cod, shrimp, sardines, and salmon -- is a great way to meet iodine needs.

When it comes to quality, seek wild-caught fish whenever possible, since farmed fish is often contaminated with PCBs, dioxins, and other unwanted chemicals.[42]

Full-Fat and Fermented Dairy Products

First, let me state that I do not believe that everyone needs to consume dairy products to obtain calcium, but if you can tolerate them, they offer many benefits beyond minerals.

Just like any food, quality counts. Sourcing your dairy products from farmers that raise their cows on pasture (grass-fed) means the milk has higher levels of fat-soluble vitamins and lower levels of pesticide residues (because they're munching on grass, not corn and soy). Dairy products labelled "organic" are the next best option, although these animals do not necessarily consume grass, just organic feed. Of course, you only benefit from the fat-soluble vitamins if you eat the fat, so seek out full-fat dairy products.

I'd like to point out one of the fat-soluble vitamins in dairy products that's especially rare in other foods and that's vitamin K2. This vitamin is different from the other major type of vitamin K, called vitamin K1, which we find in plants. Vitamin K2 functions along with vitamin A and vitamin D to support normal mineral metabolism in the body, primarily by directing minerals to be incorporated into the right places, the bones and teeth, rather than soft tissues. As you can imagine, your baby's skeleton is forming in utero, so these nutrients in combination with calcium and other minerals are the ideal nutrient matrix to form strong bones. Women who are inadequately nourished may develop maternal osteoporosis, a condition that one study was able to reverse with vitamin K2 supplementation.[43] But the effects of vitamin K2 aren't just limited to bone health. One side benefit, especially when you have gestational diabetes, is that vitamin K2 may also increase insulin sensitivity, meaning that getting enough of this nutrient could help lower your blood sugar.[44]

Fermented dairy products contain more vitamin K2 since levels of the vitamin increase through bacterial fermentation. Speaking of which, yogurt and kefir are excellent additions to your diet because they also contain beneficial bacteria called probiotics. Maternal intake of fermented milk products has been shown to reduce eczema and allergic rhinitis in their infants.[45] Regular consumption may also reduce the risk of spontaneous preterm delivery.[46]

In the next chapter, I'll discuss alternative sources of probiotics, calcium, vitamin D, and other nutrients if you are unable to consume dairy products. If you are lactose intolerant, you may be able to eat butter, cream, full-fat Greek yogurt, and aged cheese without discomfort, since these are lower in lactose.

Summary

As you can see, real food is absolutely packed with health benefits beyond what you'll find in a prenatal vitamin! And quite a few of these nutrient-dense foods that support a healthy pregnancy are the very foods you've been told to limit. Don't be surprised if your doctor or nutritionist doesn't know this information, but feel free to share it with them!

Of course, this list highlights just a few of the most critical foods that support a healthy pregnancy. So, it goes without saying, there are numerous foods beyond this list that you should include in your diet. There may also be some supplements to consider taking, as we'll explore in the next chapter.

Chapter 6

Supplements for a Healthy Pregnancy and Normal Blood Sugar

By now you know I'm an advocate of getting your nutrients from food first before resorting to supplements. However, some nutrients are difficult to obtain in adequate amounts from food alone, especially if you're a picky eater. Many of these nutrients are absolutely crucial for your growing baby, while others may be helpful in managing your blood sugar.

So in this chapter, we'll delve into those nutrients and supplements!

Prenatal Vitamin

It seems just about every OB/GYN recommends a prenatal vitamin and for good reason. During pregnancy, many nutrient needs increase and some women are not able to meet these needs with diet alone, especially when struggling with food aversions or morning sickness. But not all prenatal vitamins are created equal, so here are a few things to keep in mind.

Look for a prenatal vitamin that's food-based, as these nutrients are much more easily absorbed and utilized by the body. If you're not taking a food-based multivitamin, at the very least, ensure that it contains the appropriate form of folate, called L-methylfolate (instead of the more common folic acid or folinic acid). Researchers estimate that 40-60% of people have reduced ability to use folic acid due to genetics and therefore require the form, L-methylfolate.[47] Luckily, food contains bioavailable forms of folate, not synthetic folic acid, so ensuring you eat plenty of green leafy vegetables, nuts, eggs, and liver a few times a week, your diet should be sufficient. As you know, folate is crucial in the prevention of neural tube defects.

Vitamin D

While a prenatal vitamin will cover most of your vitamin needs, it might not contain enough vitamin D to prevent deficiency. Vitamin D is unique in that it's the only vitamin that we make from the sun and it turns out sun exposure is our main source of this vitamin, not our diet. Sun exposure accounts for 90% of vitamin D in the body in those who do not supplement.[48]

However, there are a wide variety of factors that influence our ability to produce enough vitamin D. That may explain why rates of deficiency vary considerably across the globe. Nonetheless, studies estimate the prevalence of vitamin D deficiency in pregnant women worldwide ranges between 20-85% with rates of deficiency reaching 98% in some areas.[49,50]

If you have naturally darker skin, you're are at a 6-fold higher risk for deficiency, in part due to higher levels of melanin in the skin that inhibits vitamin D production from sun exposure.[49] So keep in mind that the darker your skin tone, the more sun exposure you'll need to meet your body's demand for vitamin D. Other factors that contribute to vitamin D deficiency are inadequate sun exposure, avoidance of sun during midday (when your ability to make vitamin D is highest), inability to produce vitamin D from the sun in the winter in regions far from the equator (>33 degrees North or South), use of sunscreen, and wearing protective clothing.

The Institute for Medicine sets the dietary reference intake (DRI) for vitamin D at 600 IU/day; however, several studies have found this level of intake to be insufficient to maintain normal vitamin D levels throughout pregnancy.[51,52] Vitamin D deficiency during pregnancy puts you at higher risk for preeclampsia, low birth weight infants, and of course, gestational diabetes (according to two major meta analyses).[53,54] Vitamin D is known to impact blood sugar

70

regulation, so it comes as no surprise that early pregnancy vitamin D deficiency has been linked to a significantly increased risk for gestational diabetes.[55]

Even in women with diagnosed GD, deficiency of vitamin D may impact blood sugar control. An observational study in women with GD found that those with normal vitamin D levels had significantly lower fasting blood sugar (mean 7.2mg/dl lower), one hour post-meal blood sugar (mean 43.2mg/dl lower), and HbA1c levels (0.4% lower) compared to women with low vitamin D levels.[56] That degree of improvement is enough to prevent a woman from needing insulin or medication to manage her blood sugar.

Aside from its role in blood sugar metabolism, adequate maternal vitamin D is of crucial importance to the developing fetus. In infants with rickets (a disorder that leads to soft, weak bones), 81% of mothers had severe vitamin D deficiency while pregnant (<10ng/ml).[57] Even more concerning is the long-term impact on the health of a child born to a mother with vitamin D deficiency. A 2006 study from *The Lancet* found that bone development remained hindered at age 9 in children of mothers who were vitamin D deficient during their pregnancies.[58] Maternal vitamin D deficiency may also be associated with childhood risk of asthma, language impairment, schizophrenia, type 1 diabetes, and multiple sclerosis.[59,60,61,62,63,64]

The question then remains: How much vitamin D do expectant moms need and how do we ensure they get enough?

A recent well-designed study helped to answer this question. This was a double-blind, placebo-controlled, randomized controlled trial on vitamin D supplementation in 450 women that tested three levels of supplementation: 400 IU, 2,000 IU, and 4,000 IU per day. Their serum vitamin D levels were measured throughout pregnancy and at birth.

Supplementing with vitamin D at higher doses was not only safe, but significantly more effective at raising blood levels of vitamin D in both mother and baby.[65] Only 50% percent of women receiving 400 IU/day had sufficient serum vitamin D levels at birth, compared to 70.8% and 82.0% in the 2,000 IU and 4,000 IU groups, respectively. A similar pattern was seen in infant vitamin D sufficiency with 39.7%, 58.2% and 78.6% achieving normal vitamin D levels at birth in the 400 IU, 2,000IU, and 4,000 IU groups, respectively.

Despite supplementing with levels well above the DRI, no single adverse event was linked to vitamin D supplementation or circulating vitamin D levels and no participants experienced excessive blood levels of vitamin D. Moreover, women receiving higher doses of vitamin D supplements had significantly lower rates of pregnancy complications, including gestational diabetes. In light of the staggering rates of deficiency and the safety of supplementing with vitamin D, I believe all pregnant women should be screened for vitamin D deficiency.

Unfortunately, the American Congress of Obstetricians and Gynecologists isn't on board with universal screening. They suggest pregnant women should be screened for vitamin D deficiency *only* if they are ethnic minorities, live in cold climates, reside in northern latitudes, wear sunscreen or protective clothing, or are vegetarian.[66] However, when you know that at least two-thirds of the United States is above the 33 degree North parallel (denoted roughly by drawing a line from Long Beach, CA to Atlanta, GA), you recognize that most American women are living at a latitude where they are unable to produce enough (or any) vitamin D from sun exposure during the winter.

If your doctor has not already checked your vitamin D levels, request this simple lab test at your next visit. Normal blood levels of vitamin D are 30ng/ml or higher, although some experts suggest optimal vitamin D levels are at least 50ng/ml. Keep in mind that most prenatal vitamins only contain 400 to 600 IU of vitamin D, which simply isn't enough to keep your vitamin D at normal levels without regular midday sun exposure.

Omega-3 Fats and Fish Oil

I discussed the omega-3 fatty acids in the last chapter when referring to a few food sources, but since these fats are so crucial, they're worth exploring in a little more detail.

Most moms have heard about the benefits of omega-3 fats on brain development during pregnancy, but few know how to get enough in their diet. Some are taking additional flax seeds or chia seeds to get their omega-3 and while these are healthy for other reasons, they are *not* going to boost your baby's brain development. That's because plant-sourced omega-3s come in a form called "ALA" and the type our brain and eyes need is "DHA."

Some argue that your body can make DHA from these plant sources, but these claims don't stand up to science. It turns out the conversion of ALA to DHA in humans is incredibly poor, at most 3.8%. Plus, if your diet is high in omega-6 (which happen to be concentrated in seeds, nuts, and vegetable oils), this conversion rate drops to 1.9%.[67] A diet high in saturated fat improves this conversion rate, but the truth is: no matter what, you cannot provide enough DHA for your growing baby if you do not eat DHA directly.

Why is DHA so important? DHA is incorporated into the rapidly developing brain and eyes of the fetus during pregnancy where it assists with the formation of neurons (brain cells) and protects the brain from inflammation and damage.[68] It remains crucially important during the first two years of infancy.

The best sources of DHA are fatty fish such as salmon, herring, and sardines. DHA is also found in eggs from pastured chickens, and from the fatty meat, organs, and dairy obtained from grass-fed, pasture-raised animals. Algae is the only vegetarian source of DHA, but concentration of DHA varies considerably species to species. Some women also supplement with fish oil, cod liver oil, krill oil, or algae oil if they dislike any of the above food sources.

Ideally, you should consume a minimum of 300mg of DHA per day to provide enough for yourself and your baby. Wild Alaskan Sockeye salmon, one of the most concentrated sources of DHA, contains a whopping 1200mg in only three ounces (much more than other types of salmon). Just 2-3 meals of wild-caught salmon, sardines or other oily fish throughout the week, together with regular consumption of pastured eggs and grass-fed beef, will easily meet your needs.

Probiotics

You may already be aware of probiotics, also called "good bacteria," that live within our body and are found in fermented foods, like yogurt and kefir. It might seem strange to focus so much on bacteria, but it turns out that bacteria outnumber human cells ten-to-one in our bodies. Think about that for a minute. We are made of more bacterial cells than we are human cells (fully 90%), so it behooves us to pay attention to them.

The bacteria levels in our body are always in a state of flux based on what we eat, how we sleep, our stress levels, and more. But although most of these bacteria live in our gut, probiotics impact a lot more than digestive health. For example, it's estimated that up to 80% of our immune system is actually located in our digestive system.

New research has shown that the placenta, previously believed to be sterile, is rich with bacteria that are transferred to the developing baby throughout gestation.[69] Prior to this, we believed an infant's first contact with bacteria was through the birth canal. It has recently been shown that exposure to antibiotics during the second and third trimester, which alters bacteria levels in the body, increases a child's risk of obesity by 84%.[70] The implications of this research are not yet known, but it highlights the importance of supporting healthy bacteria levels in your body during pregnancy.

Probiotics may also influence blood sugar levels and the risk for a large baby. One study found that probiotic supplements taken during pregnancy reduced the risk of gestational diabetes up to 23% and even lowered the risk of larger babies in women with gestational diabetes.[71]

One way to ensure your body has a healthy balance of bacteria is to regularly consume fermented foods. Kefir, yogurt, and aged cheese are one source, but if you cannot tolerate dairy products there are other options. You can obtain similar benefits from raw sauerkraut, kimchi, lacto-fermented vegetables (like pickles), raw apple cider vinegar, fermented beverages (water kefir or small amounts of kombucha), miso, and natto.

It's also important to eat a wide variety of foods that contain *prebiotic* fibers, which serve as a food source to these bacteria and sustain their populations. That includes eating fiber-rich foods like vegetables, nuts, seeds, coconut, and high-fiber fruits (like berries). Limiting added sugars and refined carbohydrates also fosters the growth of healthy bacteria rather than harmful ones. This can help prevent bacterial vaginosis and yeast infections.[72]

Should you choose to supplement with probiotics, find a product that contains at least 30 billion CFUs of bacteria per serving. That might sound like a lot, but keep in mind you have over 100 trillion bacterial cells in your body, so when you see a product boasting "1 billion CFU per serving," it's like putting a drop of fresh water in a gallon of ocean water and expecting it to significantly change the saltiness. Good quality probiotic supplements will list the individual strains and the quantities of each strain on the label. Look for one that contain both *Lactobacilllus* and *Bifidus* strains.

Chia Seeds

After reading the section on omega-3 fats, you might think I wouldn't recommend chia seeds. Although they cannot provide you with DHA, chia seeds are an excellent addition to a prenatal diet for other reasons. First, because they are rich in minerals including calcium, magnesium, iron, and potassium. Secondly, they are loaded with fiber. I chose to include them in this section because chia seeds are often used like a supplement to aid digestion and blood sugar control.

Chia seeds are unique in that they have an ideal balance of soluble to insoluble fiber, meaning they can help regulate bowel movements whether you tend towards constipation or diarrhea. These fibers also serve as prebiotics, which help maintain healthy bacteria levels in the intestines. You'll notice that when chia seeds come in contact with water they release a clear gel around the seed. This gel holds onto water during intestinal transit, which is how it helps to normalize digestion and stool consistency.

Chia "gel" also slows how quickly carbohydrates are digested and absorbed, thereby regulating blood sugar. Some women take 1 tablespoon mixed into a small glass of water before meals to reduce their post-meal blood sugar, although it doesn't work for everyone.

When taking chia seeds, start with a small amount, like 1 teaspoon, and work your way up to 1-2 tablespoons per day. They do not need to be ground into a powder to be digested, unlike flaxseeds, so you can use them whole. Of course, you can use ground chia seeds if you prefer. Just be sure to store them in the refrigerator or freezer, since they contain fats that easily go rancid.

How to Use Chia Seeds:
- Chia Gel – mix 1 Tablespoon with 8oz of water, let sit for at least 5 minutes and drink
- Add to protein shakes, smoothies, or any drink
- Mix into yogurt, applesauce, unsweetened almond milk (to make "chia pudding"), etc...

Calcium

Rarely do I recommend a calcium supplement, even during pregnancy, but because this is a common question, I'll address it here.

An analysis on calcium intake in Americans (eating a standard American diet) found women aged 19-30 years consume, on average, 838mg of calcium from food alone. This number is even higher in women over 30.[73] The recommended intake for pregnancy is 1000mg, so you certainly do not need an additional high-dose calcium supplement to reach your needs. I find most women easily meet this goal when they consume a nutrient-dense real food diet as outlined in this book.

What I see more often than low calcium intake is inadequate consumption of complementary nutrients, such as vitamin D, vitamin K2, and magnesium. These nutrients are required for your body to optimally process calcium and build strong bones.

However, some women may need to pay careful attention to their calcium intake, particularly those who do not consume dairy products. Luckily, there are many non-dairy calcium sources including green leafy vegetables, bok choy, broccoli, almonds, sesame seeds, bone broth, and sardines canned with the bones. Unless you are averse to all of these foods or have another medical issue that necessitates supplementation, skip the calcium supplement.

Magnesium

Unlike calcium, magnesium deficiency is quite common. In fact, by the most recent estimates, 48% of Americans consume inadequate magnesium from food.[74] Magnesium deficiency is even more common during pregnancy and research has found that magnesium depletion, especially in the presence of calcium excess, can predispose women to vascular complications of pregnancy. Women with gestational diabetes are more likely than the average pregnant woman to be deficient in magnesium.[75]

This is a crucial finding because this mineral is a cofactor in hundreds of enzymatic reactions within the body, including those that impact blood sugar regulation. Studies on magnesium suggest that it may protect against type 2 diabetes, particularly in overweight women, so we would expect similar glycemic benefits in women with gestational diabetes.[76]

Your best food sources of magnesium are seaweed, green leafy vegetables, pumpkin seeds, Brazil nuts, sunflower seeds, sesame seeds, almonds, cashews, chia seeds, avocados, cocoa (unsweetened), bone broth, and green herbs including chives, cilantro, parsley, mint, dill, sage, and basil. However, the widespread use of aggressive farming practices, such as heavy pesticide application, has depleted the soil of magnesium. As a result, food grown in these soils is often magnesium-deficient. Organic and biodynamic farms typically have higher magnesium in the soil which is then taken up by the crops, so when possible, source your food from small farms where attention is placed on soil fertility.[77]

You can also absorb a significant amount of magnesium through your skin by soaking in Epsom salt baths or doing Epsom salt foot soaks. If you take magnesium as a supplement (orally), be aware that a common side effect is diarrhea, so start at a low dose, such as 100mg, and gradually increase to up to 300mg per day. The form of magnesium you take matters, with magnesium glycinate being one of the best absorbed forms.

One side effect of magnesium deficiency is nausea, and anecdotally some women have noticed less morning sickness when supplementing with magnesium or eating more magnesium-rich foods.

Summary
Now that you have all the information about what you put in your body, including foods and supplements, let's explore how moving your body can impact your pregnancy. The next

78

chapter will review how exercise and movement can benefit your pregnancy and your blood sugar.

Bethany's Story

When I was pregnant with my fourth child, I found out that I had gestational diabetes. I had not previously had this problem, but I think years of damage from eating a very high carb diet was finally catching up to me, even though I was not overweight. At the time, I didn't even know what a "carb" was, or that it even had any effect on my body.

I was told that I would have to bring my blood sugar levels down, or I would have to take insulin shots every day. I went to the dietitian and was instructed to eat at least 140 grams of carbohydrates per day in order to keep my sugar under control and given pamphlets with the American Diabetes Association's standard diet information.

I went on the recommended diet and tested my blood sugar about 4-5 times each day. My blood sugar would skyrocket after each meal. It was not uncommon to see it being 185-195mg/dl two hours after eating a meal. I tried exercising after eating these meals, but my sugar wouldn't go below 140mg/dl. And my morning sugar level was also high.

After a week of trying on the recommended diet (and exercising daily) I felt like a failure. I realized that the diet I was given was not helping me, so I decided to do some research. I researched day and night. Finally, I realized that I needed to eat fewer carbs in order to control my blood sugar. (Seems so simple and obvious, but it wasn't at the time).

I found a low carb, no sugar diet online. The first week was very hard. I thought I was going to die because I was so exhausted and miserable, and all I wanted was SUGAR! But, I was desperate not to go on insulin, so I stuck with it.

After a week though, it wasn't as bad and the cravings went down a lot. Plus, my blood sugar levels were dropping! I would check my blood sugar level about 10 -12 times a day, and eventually ran out of my prescription strips before it was time.

So I bought my own, and continued testing as many times as I wanted. I really wanted to know the effect of each and every food on my body.

My doctor was very impressed that I was keeping my sugar levels down. My fasting levels were the most difficult to lower, but it helped when I exercised at night and stayed away from processed carbs and sugar. In the daytime, it was easy to keep them down with diet and exercise. She encouraged me to keep up the good work, whatever I was doing. As long as my blood sugar remained under the limits she recommended, I would not have to take insulin shots.

After a few months of being on this diet, I went into labor at 38 weeks, and naturally delivered a very healthy baby boy, who is now 4 years old! Also, I lost *all* my baby weight almost immediately, and there was no "baby belly" at all. I was dumbfounded at this, because all of my previous pregnancies left me with a "baby belly", and my belly was now FLAT! What a wonderful side effect of a low carb diet!

Since then, I have been pregnant two more times. The second gestational diabetes pregnancy went well, just as the one before, and I ended up delivering a healthy 8 pound 10 ounce girl at 38 weeks. She is now 3!

On my third pregnancy with gestational diabetes, I had a new doctor who was not nearly as supportive of a low carb, high fat diet. He argued with me about it, saying my baby could end up with brain damage because I had ketones in my urine and that I would be foolish to continue it. He told me to eat more carbs and to just use metformin to bring my sugar levels down (metformin made me throw up, so I was unable to continue taking it). He asked me to keep a food log and report back to him and when he saw all the low-carb meals, he was not happy. He said my numbers were doing better, but at what cost?

Now, I don't recommend others following in my footsteps here (because I don't know how different doctors would react), but staying low carb was a choice I decided to make.

I ended up having a homebirth with my third gestational diabetes baby. He was 8 pounds even, and was very healthy. I checked his blood sugar at birth and it was perfect. I felt so energetic after having him, and never had any pain after it was over.

Let me contrast this with my first three pregnancies. I began my first pregnancy at 118 pounds, and the doctors encouraged me to gain as much weight as possible, because I was underweight.

I followed their advice. Month after month they said, "Keep gaining!" and so I did. Every morning I would have something like biscuits and gravy or cinnamon buns. For lunch I would have things like spaghetti and meatballs, lasagna, or rice stir fry. For snacks I would have cookies, brownies, or homemade bread (I thought I was eating healthy too, by the way).

I ended up gaining 60 pounds during that pregnancy. I loved having life growing inside of me, but I felt sick, tired, and miserable throughout it all. I had SEVERE heartburn every day (which I never had during my low carb pregnancies).

The doctors told me I needed to induce at 38 weeks because I had a big baby, and had a 48-hour labor with Pitocin. My baby was 8 pounds and 10 ounces. He had jaundice and had to stay overnight with bilirubin lights. I had a lot of pain in my back for about a month after he was born. I also had sciatica and had to use crutches for a while.

Then, I had *50 pounds* left to lose after he was born. I looked like I was 9 months pregnant for months after he was born. It took me 2 years to lose the weight, even with regular exercise, probably because I kept eating a high carb diet.

With my second and third pregnancy, I was determined not to gain as much weight. I gained 25 pounds with each of those, and while the babies were healthy, my labors were long, painful, and recovery was slow compared to my low carb pregnancies.

I am actually grateful that I had gestational diabetes, so that I could learn about the low carb diet and help myself through what I eat. I hope my story will inspire others to try a low carb diet as they go through their pregnancies.

Chapter 7

Prenatal Exercise

We all know exercise is healthy but somehow this becomes a controversial topic for pregnant women. In years past, expecting moms engaged in the exact same activities while pregnant as they did preconception. And while there are some considerations and adjustments to make, particularly during the final months of pregnancy, exercise is generally a very good thing!

The American Congress of Obstetricians and Gynecologists (ACOG), which provides professional guidelines for OB/GYNs across the United States, suggests pregnant women "engage in 30 minutes or more of moderate exercise on most, if not all, days of the week" unless they have medical contraindications. Despite this recommendation, pregnant women tend to reduce the duration and intensity of exercise over the course of their pregnancy.[78] This is especially undesirable for women with gestational diabetes, because exercise can help lower blood sugar.

Making matters worse, only half of physicians recommend physical activity to pregnant patients even though evidence does not suggest exercise is harmful to pregnant women or their fetus.[79] In fact, the opposite is true.

Benefits

Maternal Benefits of Exercise

Exercise during pregnancy can increase lean body mass while reducing body fat. It also strengthens the pelvic floor and improves aerobic capacity, both of which may help with labor.[80] Women who exercise regularly tend to have shorter labors and lower rates of C-sections.[81]

Beyond the physical benefits, exercise has mental and emotional effects as well, helping to relieve stress, anxiety, and depression.[81] Exercise makes it easier to stay in-tune with your body as it changes throughout the pregnancy. This mind-body awareness can help you choose exercises that help prevent lower back pain, reduce hunching in the shoulders, and reduce the chance of injury.

In general, women who exercise during their pregnancies are more likely to return to regular exercise postpartum. Since postpartum weight loss is a strong predictor of whether or not women will develop type 2 diabetes later in life, exercise becomes a useful tool in returning to preconception weight and maintaining healthy blood sugar long term.[81]

Fetal Benefits of Exercise

Children of moms who exercised during their pregnancy have a decreased risk of obesity, type 2 diabetes and metabolic syndrome[82] as well as improved oral skills and academic performance later in childhood.[83]

Researchers agree that the benefits outweigh the risks when it comes to exercise during pregnancy. The American Congress of Obstetricians and Gynecologists put out a statement in 2006 stating "concerns about maternal physical activity are not warranted," and yet I regularly hear from clients that they are afraid to exercise because they might "hurt the baby."

To put it into perspective, think of it this way. The increased circulation from exercise is a good thing, as it brings new blood, nutrients, and oxygen to your fetus. Remember, the only way your baby is getting nourishment and excreting waste is through your circulation. Keep that blood moving!

Benefits of Exercise for Gestational Diabetes

When it comes to gestational diabetes, exercise plays a major role in blood sugar control. Exercise reduces fasting blood sugar, post-meal blood sugar (especially when performed after a meal), increases insulin sensitivity, and reduces the need for medication and insulin.[84]

In general, women who exercise throughout their pregnancy gain less weight. This is crucial because a major complication of gestational diabetes is macrosomia (large birth weight) and aside from blood sugar, maternal weight gain plays a major role in the weight of your baby at birth.[85] Increased birth weight is linked to childhood overweight and other health problems. In women who are not yet diagnosed with gestational diabetes, exercise may actually reduce the risk by 49-78%.[86]

Starting an Exercise Program

The ideal exercise program for women varies based on individual abilities, preferences and fitness level before pregnancy. In general, aim for 30 minutes of exercise every day, including both strength and aerobic exercise.

Goals for exercise include achieving medical targets like maintaining normal blood sugar and blood pressure, but should also take into consideration the type of activity you actually *like* to do. It's about making the pregnancy easier and healthier, not punishing yourself.

If you're not used to exercising, start slow, such as adding a 10 minute walk after lunch. Once that becomes easy, you can gradually add on until you reach 30 minutes of movement in total over the course of the day, keeping in mind you can exercise for longer if it feels good. Some women choose to break this 30 minutes into shorter stints. For some, a 10 minute walk after each meal gives them better glycemic control. Others like to do 30 minutes of exercise in one go. It's up to you, how your body feels, and how your blood sugar responds.

If you do not already exercise, be sure to check with your doctor to rule out any specific contraindications or situations in which exercise should be avoided.

Considerations if You Take Insulin or Medication

Since insulin and glyburide both have risks of hypoglycemia (low blood sugar), be sure to talk to your healthcare provider before engaging in exercise if you are taking one or both of those medicines. Timing your exercise consistently at a certain part of the day may be the best way to keep your blood sugar within normal range (rather than exercising in the morning some days and late evening other days).

Be aware that since blood sugar tends to go down with exercise, you may need to adjust the timing and/or dose of your medicine. Exercising immediately after a meal or snack reduces the risk of hypoglycemia. Pay close attention to your energy levels and always have your blood glucose meter, water, and an emergency carbohydrate-containing snack handy. Refer to the moderate carb snacks in Chapter 4.

If you are taking metformin, which has virtually no risk of hypoglycemia, or if you are not taking any blood sugar medications, these hypoglycemia concerns do not apply. Simply exercise after a meal or snack and stay hydrated. Of course, if you feel low energy or have other symptoms of hypoglycemia, test your blood sugar to confirm.

Precautions for Pregnancy

There are some considerations pregnant women should take to make sure the exercise regimen they choose is safe and effective. Once you have your doctor's approval, there are a few things to keep in mind.

First is to become aware that your body is going through amazing and necessary changes to accommodate your growing baby. Pregnancy causes an increase in blood volume, cardiac output and respiratory rate, which may make it feel like it's hard to catch your breath. In the third trimester, this is compounded by the fact that baby is larger and pressing up into your lungs, thus limiting your lung capacity (and therefore oxygen intake). Listen to your body and use the "talk test," described below, to asses your efforts and limits.

Heart Rate

Many women want to check their heart rate to monitor their body during exercise, but since heart rate does not correlate with exertion during pregnancy, it's not recommended as a reliable measure, nor is there a set guideline on what heart rate is ideal or too high during pregnancy.[81]

In general, the fear is that if you exercise too hard, your body will divert blood flow from the placenta to working muscles, which would result in heart rate changes in the fetus. This however, is not the case. Moderately strenuous exercise does not induce fetal distress or decrease fetal heart rate in healthy pregnant women.[87] Rest assured, moderate aerobic activity throughout your pregnancy is beneficial and can even increase your endurance, making labor easier.

Talk Test

If you're having trouble breathing, can't catch your breath, or are unable to say a short sentence, you are exercising too hard. Slow down and catch your breath. An increase in heart rate and respiration is fine, just not to the point where you cannot get enough oxygen or feel faint. A good level to be at is a noticeable increase in heart rate while still being able to carry on a light conversation. I realize this advice is vague; however, the "talk test" correlates better to exertion during pregnancy than any other measure.[88]

Don't Over-Stretch

During pregnancy your body releases a hormone called relaxin, which as the name suggests, helps *relax* your ligaments. Without relaxin, your pelvis would not be able to open and allow you to birth your baby vaginally! It's actually a pretty neat system when you think about it.

The only downside is to this is that ligaments can become a little *too* loose leading to joint instability and pain, especially in the pubic symphysis (pubic bone) and sacroiliac joints (very low back and hips). This makes activities like jumping, twists and turns with sudden starts or stops potentially problematic. Use caution with stretching and yoga, especially in the third trimester when you're carrying around the extra weight of your baby (and of course, your placenta, amniotic fluid, etc.). Know your limits and don't push it.

Also keep in mind that higher impact activities, including running, may become uncomfortable. Prenatal weight gain can increase forces on the knees and hips as much as 100% during events like running. If you were running regularly prior to conception, it's generally considered safe to continue during pregnancy, but *do* listen to your body. If it becomes uncomfortable, opt for lower impact activities like walking, swimming, moderate hiking or using an elliptical machine. Lower impact aerobics ease stress on those joints. With any physical discomfort from exercise, it's wise to *not* "work through the pain."

Posture, Alignment, and Back Pain
Exercise is only beneficial and safe if you do it with good form. This is even more important during pregnancy, when your body has to cope with a shift in your center of gravity. As your belly grows, it pulls your weight forward. Many women tend to jut their hips forward (and lean back) in an attempt to counterbalance the weight of their baby, but this causes overarching and compression in the lower back. That, along with looser joints, are the major culprits in lower back pain.

Instead of allowing the weight of the baby to pull you forward, use your abdominal muscles to draw your navel towards your spine while you simultaneously get taller (by imagining a string pulling you up from the crown of your head). With proper alignment, your head should be directly over your shoulders, shoulders centered over your rib cage, rib cage centered over your hips, hips over your knees, knees over your ankles, and weight evenly distributed between the balls of the feet and the heels. It's a lot to think about!

If your breasts have grown or if you're not conscious of your posture, you may also experience upper back pain, as your shoulders begin to hunch forward and close in towards your chest. Practice stretching "open" your chest and strengthen the muscles of the upper back (between the shoulder blades) to offset this tendency. Imagine your collar bones lifting up away from your belly and pulling apart towards the sides of your body.

Back pain is compounded when abdominal muscles are weak, since the abdominal muscles help you maintain alignment and "lift" in your spine. Later I'll review some sample exercises to help you with this.

Abdominal, Back, and Pelvic Floor Strength

In addition to my nutrition background, I'm also a certified Pilates instructor, and I've taught Pilates to many women throughout their pregnancies and postpartum. I've repeatedly observed, firsthand, its beneficial effects on strength, stabilization, and flexibility. Pilates is an excellent option for expecting moms because it combines aerobic and strength exercise into one workout. It also works within the normal range of motion for joints and strengthens small stabilizing muscles, thus reducing the risk of overstretching ligaments that is so common in pregnant women.

Pilates focuses attention on the abdominal, back, and pelvic floor muscles, which all tend to get weak during pregnancy. And yet, it is these muscles that are critical in maintaining healthy posture and vaginally birthing a baby!

PROPER ALIGNMENT

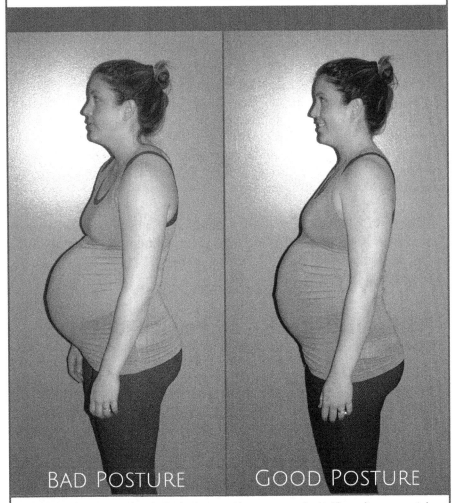

BAD POSTURE   GOOD POSTURE

The above photos are taken just minutes apart in a woman who is 40 weeks pregnant. In the example of "bad posture", notice the arching in her lower back and the tilt of her pelvis as she allows the weight of the baby to pull her forward. Also, note how her shoulders and upper back are hunched, causing her head to jut forward and strain her neck.

In the example of "good posture", she uses her abdominal and back muscles to lift and hold the baby close to her spine. This aligns her spine, reducing compression and pain in the lower back and neck. She has lengthened her spine, lifted her ribcage, and very literally created space for the baby in her torso. Also notice the length in her neck, the openness in her chest, and the position of her head directly over her shoulders.

Note on Abdominal Exercises

Many doctors warn against abdominal exercise during pregnancy, citing an increased risk of diastasis recti, in which the rectus abdominus ("6-pack" muscles that run vertically from lower ribs to pubic bone) separate at the center, leaving a gap. Diastasis recti, however, should not occur from abdominal exercises unless you are engaging the wrong muscles.

Before starting any and *every* abdominal movement, pregnant or not (and even when getting out of bed), you should draw your navel towards your spine, then draw your navel up towards your rib cage. This engages the tranversus abdominus ("corset" muscles), the deep muscles in the lower back, and the muscles of the pelvic floor, thereby preventing the rectus abdominus from trying to do all the work.

You can tell you're doing it right if you lay on your back and attempt to do a crunch. If your belly bulges out as if you have a 2x4 coming out of your abdomen (some call this "tenting"), you're not pulling your navel "in and up" enough. If instead your belly stays relatively the same size as you lift your head and you don't observe any "tenting" of the abdominal muscles, you're now engaging the appropriate muscles and not over-utilizing the rectus abdominus. Good job, mama!

Sample Exercises

Hip Stabilization

Lay on your back. Put your hands on the pointy part of your hip bones. Imagine a rubber band hooked between the hip bones. From the inside, imagine tightening that rubber band and bringing your hip bones closer together, using your muscles to pull your hip bones towards the center line of your body. Hold for 10 seconds. Release all muscle tension with a few deep breaths. Repeat 5-10 times.

Abdominal Exercises

Abdominal exercises reduce the risk of back injury and strain. All of the sample exercises here should be done while engaging the abdominal muscles, but this simple exercise specifically targets those muscles while also strengthening the low back. But don't think simple means easy! If you're not shaking, you're not doing this right.

Sit on a cushy mat with your knees bent, feet on the floor. Sit up as tall as you can and draw your navel to your spine and draw your lowest ribs backwards slightly (without changing your posture). Bring the arms straight in front of you. Lean back about 30 degrees while maintaining a lifted spine. Do not let the low back "sink" down. Hold for a count of 10-15 seconds. Return to the starting position. Repeat 3-5 times.

You can progress this exercise by lifting the arms, opening the arms wide, or by making arm circles (try one at a time to challenge your obliques). Play around and have fun. You can also lean back further when you've developed the strength to do so without compromising your form.

Squats
Stand with your feet slightly wider than hips distance apart. Engage your core muscles. Bend your knees and squat down letting your butt stick out behind you. Keep your spine straight (not arched or rounded). Return to standing. Repeat 10-20 times. Bend as low as is comfortable for your knees. You may lift the arms as you squat to stay balanced. Add light weights and change up the arm movements if you want more of a challenge.

Cat & Cow Stretch
Start on your hands and knees with hands shoulder distance apart and knees hip distance apart. Ensure your hips are right over your knees and shoulders are right over your wrists, gently pulled away from your ears. Start with a flat back. Take an inhale. Exhale as you round your back by pulling your belly button towards your spine and moving your ribs towards the ceiling. Let your head drop. Inhale as you reverse your spine allowing the belly to relax and the chest to open up. Lift your gaze slightly without craning the neck too much. Repeat 5-10 times.

Child's Pose

Kneel and sit back on your heels. Open up your knees wide. Place your hands on the floor in front of you and gently lean forward until your belly is resting between the knees. You can place your hands in front of the body and gently push into the floor to better stretch your back. Or you may choose to rest here and release all muscle tension.

Side Lying Chest Opener

This stretch is great first thing in the morning when still lying in bed.

Lie on your side with your knees pulled towards your chest and your hands behind your head. Leaving your hands behind your head, bring your elbows together until they touch. Inhale as you open up the chest and allow the "top" elbow to draw towards the ceiling and behind the body. Pause to feel the stretch. Exhale as you return to the starting position. For a more intense stretch, ensure that your knees stay together as you open up the chest. Repeat 5-10 times on each side.

Side Leg Series: Circles, Lifts, Point Flex

Lie on your side with your legs straight at a 45 degree angle (slightly in front of your body). Use your bottom arm to prop up your head. Your other arm can rest on the mat to stabilize you. Position yourself so your hips are stacked on top of one another. Engage your abdominal muscles to stabilize your body. Imagine your top leg is longer than your bottom leg.
This series should be completed on both sides.

Circles

Begin by lifting the top leg to hip level and make small circles 10 times in each direction. Ensure that only the top leg is moving and the rest of your body is completely still. This requires strong engagement of the abdominal and oblique muscles.

Lifts

Lift the top leg about 2 feet from the bottom leg. Hold for a count of 3. Lower down. Repeat 5x.

Point/Flex

This is exactly like the "lifts" exercise above. This time point your foot before you lift the leg, then flex the foot as you lower the leg down. Repeat 3-5x. Then reverse the movement and flex the foot as you lift it up, then point as you lower down.

Wall Push Ups

There are 2 version of this exercise: Regular Push-ups and Tricep Push-ups. If you are used to doing push-ups, you can do these on the floor or on your knees (instead of against a wall).

Regular Push-ups

Stand 1-2 feet away from the wall with your feet parallel and hip distance apart. Lift your heels 2 inches off the ground. Place your hands on the wall directly in front of your shoulders. Spread your hands about 2 feet apart. Do 10 push-ups, keeping your body in a straight line.

Tricep Push-ups

Place your hands on the wall directly in front of your shoulders, only about 1 foot apart. Bring your body towards the wall by bending your elbows, keeping them close to your body. Repeat 10 times.

Plank

Begin in a push-up position on the floor. You can choose to do this on your feet or on your knees. If you have wrist issues, you can do this on your elbows (although that becomes more difficult later in pregnancy when your belly has grown).

Place your hands on the floor shoulder distance apart. Come into a push-up position. Ensure your wrists are directly under your shoulders. Keep your body in a straight line. Push energy through your hands into the floor to engage the muscles of the upper back. Ensure your abdominal muscles are pulled in to protect your lower back. Hold for 20-60 seconds. Rest and repeat 2-5 times.

Adjusting Exercise by Trimester

First Trimester
In general, there are no major changes you should make to your exercise regimen other than avoiding the usual activities that jerk, bounce or risk abdominal injury. You may experience more fatigue or nausea during the first trimester, so if your body does not allow you to exercise, don't worry. Many women have a boost in energy in the second and third trimester. Do stay open to the possibility that a short 5-15 minute walk might help you feel better. Or consider practicing gentle yoga or a short series of Pilates exercises, such as the side-lying leg series.

Second Trimester
Exercises done lying on your back may become uncomfortable at this stage in pregnancy, depending on how much weight you have gained. This is because your baby's weight is pressing on the vena cava, a large vein that carries blood from the lower extremities back to the heart. This can make it difficult for you to receive enough blood and oxygen, leaving you light headed. There's no long term harm if you experience this. Simply sit up, catch your breath, and make note of what you experienced. Take care to avoid lying on your back for long periods of time.

For this same reason, exercises where the hips go above your heart -- such as bridge pose in yoga, pelvic tilts in Pilates, or any inversions -- are generally avoided beyond 16 weeks. The exact timing, again, will depend on how much weight you have gained and other factors, so simply pay close attention to your symptoms and your body, modifying exercises for comfort.

In general, short bursts of activity performed lying on your back, such as a series of abdominal exercises, are fine, depending on your symptoms. Some women will choose to prop themselves up at a slight angle with pillows, blankets, or bolsters for those activities.

Third Trimester

In the third trimester, increased joint laxity becomes more obvious as you're now carrying more weight from your growing baby and uterus. Take care to avoid over-stretching. Participating in joint stabilizing exercises, such as Pilates, can help you cope with this.

Make good posture a priority. Regularly reassess your posture and sit up straight, with shoulders gently pulled back and your chest open.

Your growing baby is also likely pushing up on your lungs, making it harder to catch your breath. Adjust the intensity of exercises as needed, being sure to never get too out of breath (remember the "talk test"). Baby is also compressing your stomach, so avoid large meals immediately before exercising.

At this stage you are also more likely to become overheated, so take rests when exercising to cool down and hydrate. Avoid exercising outside during hot or humid weather.

The third trimester is also the most common time for you to experience Braxton Hicks contractions, the unpredictable, but usually not painful, "practice" contractions that many healthcare providers believe prepare and tone the uterus for actual labor. When they happen, the uterus may tighten for 30-60 seconds or longer, then taper off. They generally are non-rhythmic and irregular in intensity. If you notice slight contractions during exercise (and especially if you're far from your due date), they might be Braxton Hicks. Just stop and allow the contractions to pass before resuming your activity. If they continue or become painful, call your provider immediately. Braxton Hicks are more common when dehydrated, so be sure to always carry water with you when exercising.

Monitoring

Once you begin exercising, be sure to track how exercise affects your blood sugar. You may notice a change in your blood sugar after exercise (usually a decrease), sometimes necessitating an adjustment to the timing of snacks, meals, or medicines. The more aware you are of these effects, the more in control you are of your pregnancy.

Summary

Exercise is safe, effective, and beneficial during pregnancy. Listen to your body and healthcare provider for specific adjustments to make to your exercise routine.

For more insights on prenatal exercise, visit
www.RealFoodforGD.com.

PRENATAL EXERCISE CHEAT SHEET

Exercise 30 minutes or more every day
Include strength exercises 2-3x/week

Aerobic – walking, jogging, stairs, elliptical, dancing, swimming, stationary bike, low impact aerobics, moderate hiking
Strength – arm and leg exercises, light weights, Pilates, prenatal yoga, resistance training
Flexibility – Pilates, prenatal yoga, stretching
Abdominal/pelvic floor exercises – daily to help ease low back pain and prepare for labor. Use your muscles to "hold the baby close" to your body.

Benefits
- **Complications** – Lowers blood sugar and blood pressure, prevents excess weight gain, prevents larger than normal babies. Also reduces bloating, stretch marks, low back pain, constipation, varicose veins, swelling in legs and feet.
- **Strength** – Improves posture, muscle tone, endurance
- **Mental Health** – Boosts your mood, less stress, anxiety, depression, better sleep
- **Postpartum** – Reduces postpartum weight retention and risk of pelvic prolapse

General Guidelines
- Take frequent breaks to prevent overheating; don't exercise in hot weather
- Drink plenty of fluids to prevent dehydration
- Eat before exercising
- Wear comfortable, supportive clothing (sports bra) and shoes
- After the 4th month (16 weeks), avoid exercises lying on your back

Exercises to Avoid
Do not play contact sports. Avoid movements that jerk, bounce or risk abdominal injury: soccer, football, baseball, hockey, basketball, kickboxing, downhill skiing, gymnastics, etc.

Precautions
Check with your doctor to see if exercise is safe during your pregnancy. Exercise with a partner if you can. Talk with your healthcare team if you take insulin or blood sugar medication, since your meal plan or insulin may need to be adjusted.

Signs to Stop Exercising
If you experience the following, call your doctor:
- Contractions of the uterus
- Decreased fetal movement
- Dizziness, chest pains, headache, or shortness of breath
- Vaginal bleeding or leaking of amniotic fluid

Chapter 8

Medication Management

One of the biggest fears women have when first diagnosed with gestational diabetes is that they'll need insulin or medication. Their fear is so great that it's sometimes the primary motivator to change their diet, begin exercising, and monitor their blood sugar closely.

Often doctors or healthcare providers will pull the "unless you want insulin" card as an ultimatum to push women into taking this diagnosis more seriously. I've always felt at odds with that approach, because our goals as health practitioners and your goals as a mom are to have the healthiest pregnancy possible, nothing less. Clearly, if you're reading this book, that's true for you and you're motivated to make the necessary lifestyle changes. It also paints the picture that medication is "bad" or should be avoided at all costs, when really it's just another tool we have to manage blood sugar.

There are many factors that can influence your need for medication. Viewing medication from the stance that it's for people who "fail diet therapy," which by the way is the actual and accepted medical terminology, subtly and unfairly blames the woman for her blood sugar levels.

However, there are many factors that make controlling your blood sugar with gestational diabetes a challenge. While the majority of women *are* able to do it with diet and exercise, not everyone can. If you started this pregnancy at a higher weight or gained a lot of weight early in the pregnancy, your body is naturally more insulin resistant. Same thing if your family is of an ethnicity where diabetes is common or if there is a direct family history of diabetes (including gestational diabetes). Women who are older or have already had children tend to have more insulin resistance as well. Regardless of the above, *every* woman develops some level of insulin resistance during her pregnancy, and for some this means they are unable to keep their blood sugar controlled without a little help, particularly when it comes to fasting blood sugar.

My goal is to provide you with the most effective approach to lowering blood sugar with lifestyle without chastising the use of insulin or medication.

That being said, having worked clinically with hundreds of women with gestational diabetes and by using my nutrition approach (described in earlier chapters), which *does* sway from conventional guidelines, I've seen the need for insulin and medication drop significantly. Actually, within the first few months of working as a prenatal nutritionist and diabetes educator for one clinic, the director pulled me aside to share the dramatic improvement in our patients' progress since I came on board. It turns out the number of women who "failed diet therapy" and the number of new prescriptions for insulin and medication were *way* down. This was attributed to my excellent teaching of the gestational diabetes management class. Of course, I knew it wasn't because my teaching skills were somehow magical, but because the content and focus of that class had changed to embrace real, nutrient-dense foods and mindful eating (not the usual low-fat, high-carbohydrate, calorie-restricted nutrition recommendations).

In addition, the women who did require insulin or medication were able to normalize their blood sugars on far lower doses than were customary in this clinic. This alone provided a sharp decrease in how often our patients experienced dangerous hypoglycemia or side effects. They also didn't typically exceed their weight gain guidelines, but at the same time weren't complaining of hunger or food cravings. Our rates of macrosomia (infants born very large) and complications at birth plummeted. It really was amazing to witness.

Medical research is beginning to support this approach. One study found that "Using a low-glycemic index diet for women with GDM effectively halved the number needing to use insulin, with no compromise of obstetric or fetal outcomes."[89]

Still, for the women who do require a little medical intervention, know this: Normalizing your blood sugar with medication is far safer than "going natural" and having blood sugar outside of the natural and safe range. In fact, *any* elevation in blood sugars outside the normal range is linked to increased risk of C-sections, neonatal hypoglycemia, premature delivery, shoulder dystocia or birth injury, intensive neonatal care, jaundice, and preeclampsia according to a major and groundbreaking study of over 23,000 women called the Hyperglycemia and Adverse Pregnancy Outcomes study (HAPO) published in the highly respected *New England Journal of Medicine*.[90]

So if, despite your best efforts, your blood sugar is still coming out high and your doctor is suggesting medication or insulin, it's in your best interest to follow his or her advice.

In my personal experience, the nutritional recommendations in this book are consistently effective for post-meal blood sugar, but many women have trouble with their fasting blood sugar. If this is an issue for you and you've followed all the tips and tricks described in Chapter 9, you might need a little help. Similarly, some women may feel better eating a slightly higher carbohydrate diet that leads to higher blood sugars after meals and choose to take insulin or medication to bring those numbers to normal. And that's ok, too!

Below I'll describe the common medications used in pregnancy, possible side effects, and tips for success.

Insulin

Insulin works the same way that the naturally occurring insulin does in your body. It tells your cells to take sugar out of your bloodstream to be used for energy. Insulin is given by syringe as a shot.

As you may already know, there are many types of insulin. Only a few are approved for use during pregnancy, namely short-acting insulin and long-acting insulin. Short-acting insulin is taken before a meal to lower your blood sugar from the food you've eaten, while long-acting insulin is taken either once or twice a day and slowly releases a small amount of insulin over many hours. Depending on your unique situation and blood sugar pattern, your doctor may recommend one or both of these insulins at particular times during the day.

Tips For Success
- Regularly test your blood sugar
- Aim to eat a consistent amount of carbohydrates at each meal
- Take insulin at the exact time and in the exact dose recommended by your healthcare team
- Don't be scared if your insulin doses are increased by your doctor. It takes time to find the perfect dose for you, as every body is different. Also, as your pregnancy progresses and the placenta grows, your body becomes more insulin resistant and often necessitates higher doses of insulin. This is normal, not a sign of failure.

Possible Side Effects
If you take too much insulin or take it at the wrong time, a common side effect is low blood sugar (hypoglycemia). Symptoms include hunger, nausea, sweating or clammy skin, anxiety, nervousness, increased heart rate, mood changes, and low energy. If you experience any of these, test your blood sugar. If your blood sugar is near or less than 60mg/dl, the treatment is to consume 15 grams of carbohydrate, then retest your blood sugar in 15 minutes. (Realize that hypoglycemia is defined as less than 70mg/dl if you are not pregnant, but less than 60mg/dl when you are pregnant.)

The best treatments for hypoglycemia are snacks or drinks that contain carbohydrates along with some fat and protein, to stabilize your blood sugar and prevent another low.

Some examples:
- 8 oz whole milk + a small handful of almonds
- 1 apple + 2 tablespoons peanut butter
- 4 oz fruit juice + 2 oz cheese

If after eating one of the above snacks your blood sugar is still low, consume another snack.

Ideally, your insulin doses should be matched to your food intake, so you don't experience either highs or lows. This takes a period of adjustment, careful monitoring, and open communication with your healthcare provider. Keep a very detailed Food & Blood Sugar Log!

Myths About Insulin

One of the primary reasons women don't want to take insulin is because they believe if they take it during pregnancy, they will need it for the rest of their lives. This is untrue, but an understandable fear nonetheless. Usually when we think of insulin, we think of people with type 1 diabetes (rare) or long-standing type 2 diabetes (much more common). In these folks, their body doesn't produce insulin (or very, very little), which means they need insulin shots for the rest of their lives. And because having poorly controlled diabetes for a long time increases health risks, people associate poor health with insulin. In reality, the complications are caused by having high blood sugar for many years, not the insulin.

With gestational diabetes, your body is still producing insulin, but maybe not enough to keep your blood sugar at normal levels and overcome the insulin resistance associated with pregnancy. So, if you do need insulin shots, you'll likely only need them during the pregnancy. Once you deliver, 90% of women see their blood sugar return to normal levels as your hormone levels drop. It's actually much safer for you and your baby to take insulin (or medication) during pregnancy and have normal blood sugar than it is to go without. I'll expand more on the long-term blood sugar issues and the risk of "converting" to type 2 diabetes in Chapter 10.

Metformin

Metformin is an oral diabetes medication that has been used to treat type 2 diabetes for decades. Its use in pregnancy is more recent than insulin, but it has a few advantages. Metformin works in three ways: by increasing your body's response to its own insulin (lowering insulin resistance), reducing the amount of glucose produced by the liver, and reducing the amount of glucose absorbed from food. Because metformin does not stimulate the release of insulin from the pancreas, it has virtually no risk of causing hypoglycemia.

Not all doctors are using metformin in pregnancy; however, those that do find it to be safe, effective, and well tolerated. The primary concern is that metformin crosses the placenta; however, it has not been associated with birth defects or adverse outcomes, even when used during the first trimester of pregnancy.[91] In studies, no statistical differences between diet and metformin groups were found with regard to the rates of miscarriage, prematurity, preeclampsia, small-for-gestational-age (SGA) or large-for-gestational-age (LGA) newborns, cesarean deliveries, neonatal intensive care unit admissions, birth malformations or neonatal injuries.[92]

Some doctors even suggest that metformin may be beneficial for the infant, since it may reduce the risk of insulin resistance in the fetus.[93]

Recent studies confirm that metformin has a place in managing gestational diabetes, especially for women who are not comfortable injecting insulin or have other markers of metabolic syndrome, which include increased blood pressure, overweight, excess body fat around the waist, and abnormal cholesterol levels. "Metformin is an effective alternative to insulin in the treatment of GDM patients."[91] Some doctors choose to combine metformin with insulin therapy, as metformin can help minimize the doses of insulin by improving insulin sensitivity.

Tips For Success
Take metformin with food to minimize digestive discomfort. Also, it may take a few weeks to observe noticeable changes in your blood sugar.

Possible Side Effects

- Digestive discomfort. Initially, metformin can cause nausea, gas, bloating, or diarrhea. These symptoms are minimized when metformin is started at a low dose and increased gradually. Digestive issues usually subside within a week or so.
- Metformin can cause vitamin B12 deficiency with long-term use. I suggest supplementing with the methylcobalamin form of vitamin B12 if your prenatal vitamin does not contain it. Consuming adequate calcium reduces the risk of vitamin B12 deficiency when taking metformin.[94]
- Slowed weight gain or slight weight loss is a common, and usually welcomed, side effect. For this reason, metformin may be particularly beneficial for overweight women.

Glyburide

Glyburide is an older oral diabetes medication that works by triggering the pancreas to release more insulin. Some find this medication to be controversial. The concern is that this medication crosses the placenta in small amounts and may also stimulate the release of insulin in the fetal pancreas, potentially hyperstimulating the baby's insulin production before birth, which triggers increased deposition of abdominal fat in the fetus (and potentially alters the metabolism of the baby later in life). This, however, remains speculative, and many doctors use glyburide regularly.

Some studies suggest "therapeutic approaches should be targeted towards relieving the demand on the beta cell to secrete insulin" to preserve pancreatic function.[95] With gestational diabetes, your pancreas is already fighting an up-hill battle of hyperstimulated insulin production from the pancreas coupled with insulin resistance. Glyburide further pushes it to its limits.

That being said, studies on glyburide use during pregnancy show it's an effective alternative to insulin.[96]

Tips For Success

If you are prescribed glyburide, you may find you need to eat more carbohydrates to prevent low blood sugar. You may also need to eat more frequently, for example, every 2 hours instead of every 3 to 4 to prevent low blood sugar. You may also need to wake up in the middle of the night to have a snack if your blood sugar is dropping low while you sleep.

Possible Side Effects

- The main side effect is hypoglycemia, or low blood sugar, as I described above. Be sure to carry a carbohydrate-containing snack with you at all times if you are taking glyburide. Be conscious of the signs and symptoms of hypoglycemia as described in the insulin section and treat accordingly.
- Another side effect is increased weight gain. Since glyburide stimulates the release of insulin, regardless of which foods you eat, some women find they need to eat more food and more carbohydrates to prevent hypoglycemia. This, in turn, may lead to excess weight gain.

Summary

Whether or not you need to take medication during your pregnancy, it's helpful to be informed about the options and considerations. Remember that your nutrition and exercise choices still make a huge difference in your blood sugar, even if you need a little "boost" from medication or insulin.

Chapter 9

Help! Solutions to Common Questions and Concerns

By now you have a good understanding of gestational diabetes and the nutrition principles, exercise habits, and medications (if you need them) that help keep your blood sugar under control. But if you're human, and I sure hope you are, chances are you've run into a few snags.

This chapter will tackle some common challenges and offer solutions for you to experiment with. Remember, every body responds differently and each pregnancy is unique. So be gentle with yourself when things don't go perfectly. Hopefully this chapter will give you a little peace of mind and some direction when you need it most.

Like many things in life, gestational diabetes is a process of self discovery. Not everything here will apply to you and you may find solutions that I did not specifically mention. As always, this is not meant to replace the advice of your healthcare provider(s), so please consult them before making any changes.

My fasting blood sugar is high. What can I do?

This is a tough one, as there can be many potential causes and solutions. Since overnight blood sugar levels vary greatly, keep in mind that high fasting blood sugar could be from having high blood sugar all night, or could be a rebound reaction if your blood sugar drops too low. Confusing, I know. It's also normal for fasting blood sugar to fluctuate by 12-15% day-to-day during pregnancy, so calculate your average fasting blood sugar over the last week or two before freaking out when you get a reading of 96mg/dl one day when your usual is 84mg/dl.

To start, make sure you're checking your fasting blood sugar first thing in the morning when you naturally wake up. If you wait more than 30 minutes after waking, your blood sugar might go up as your body releases stored sugar to fuel you for the day. I suggest leaving your meter near your bedside to remind you (although, remember it's best to wash your hands before checking your blood sugar).

If you're already doing the above and still have high fasting numbers, you can start using your Food & Blood Sugar Log to figure this out. Take note of the timing of your dinner and bedtime snack (you are eating a bedtime snack, right?!). If you eat these too early and go to sleep late, your blood sugar may be dropping too low at night, setting the "emergency alarms" off. Essentially, your body may think you're starving and trigger the release of stored glucose from your liver to bring your blood sugar level up to fuel your heart, your brain, and your baby. (Remember, in a way, baby is "eating" 24/7!) Having a snack within an hour or so of going to sleep can help prevent this unwanted drop and rebound spike in blood sugar the next morning. In general, leaving no more than 10 hours between your last bite of food at night and first bite of food in the morning can prevent this.

For the same reason, sleeping in too late can also result in high fasting blood sugar. You might experiment with waking up earlier to check your sugar, even if you go back to sleep, to get a more accurate reading.

If you suspect your blood sugar is dropping too low in the middle of the night (causing the rebound high fasting blood sugar), you can set an alarm to wake up in the middle of the night to check your blood sugar. Sometimes if your blood sugar is low, you may wake up hungry in the middle of the night (though not always). It's ok to get up and eat something, but you may prevent this in the future by adding more fat and protein to your bedtime snack. This may stabilize your blood sugar overnight, so you can get a full night's sleep. For example, include one of the following options: nuts, cheese, meat, egg, or full-fat Greek yogurt.

On the flip side, if you're eating a large dinner, late at night, and going to sleep with high blood sugar, it could be staying that way while you sleep. I suggest eating one of the dinners outlined in Chapter 5 that's moderate in carbohydrates (no more than 30g), then (after checking your post-dinner blood sugar), having a snack before bedtime. If that's still not helping, you can play around with the balance of carbohydrates-to-fat-to-protein at this snack and observe your fasting blood sugar day to day.

Lastly, we know exercise has an impact on fasting blood sugar. Are you getting the recommended 30 minutes of exercise every day?

If all of the above doesn't make much difference, you might benefit from medication to help manage your fasting blood sugar. I know it seems like I'm obsessing over this number, but we know that seemingly minor elevations in fasting blood sugar are linked to big babies (macrosomia). From the Hyperglycemia and Adverse Pregnancy Outcomes study (HAPO) we know the chance of having a large baby was only 10% if fasting blood sugar was maintained at 90mg/dl average or less, but this number rose to 17% at an average of 95mg/dl, and 25-35% at an average fasting blood sugar of 100.[97]

Remember, some things are within our control and some things aren't. It's safer to have the help of medication than to risk exposing your baby to consistently high blood sugar.

I have high blood sugar after meals. Why?

First, are you monitoring your food intake? The most common cause of high blood sugar after meals is too many carbohydrates at once. Start by measuring the amount of carbohydrates at each meal and watch for trends. Use measuring cups, food labels or even meal tracking software to calculate the amount of carbohydrates at the meal. Opt for higher fiber carbohydrates when given the option, such as beans and lentils, berries, and non-starchy vegetables (or even adding a tablespoon of chia seeds with your meal). If you haven't already, eliminate foods made with white sugar and white flour.

You may also notice that if you have too many carbohydrates without balancing them with protein and fat, your blood sugar will spike. Consult the suggested meals and snacks for more detailed food suggestions. Some women have variable carbohydrate tolerance at different times of the day, as I'll explain in the next question.

My blood sugar is always high after breakfast, but normal every other time. What's going on?

Many women have trouble with high blood sugar after breakfast. Naturally, your body has a surge in cortisol and placental hormones in the morning, which makes your body more insulin resistant. This means you may be less able to handle carbohydrates at breakfast than other times of the day. That's why, if you look closely, the sample breakfast options in the meal plans included in this book limit carbohydrate intake more at breakfast than other meals. You can experiment with consuming a breakfast that has no more than 15g of carbohydrates and see if it helps. For example, you might try a small organic corn tortilla with 1-2 eggs, cheese, and fresh tomato (or any non-starchy vegetables). See the meal plans in Chapter 4 for other suggestions.

When I was first diagnosed, my blood sugar was almost always normal. Now it's usually high for no apparent reason. What am I doing wrong?

Don't blame yourself so fast! Hormone levels and insulin resistance go up in later pregnancy. For that reason some women's bodies are unable to produce enough insulin to keep their blood sugar at normal levels. There are a few things you can try to see how much you can lower your blood sugar naturally. If you have not already lowered the carbohydrates in your diet, that's the first step. Refer to Chapters 3 and 4 for nutrition guidance. If you do not already exercise regularly, you can add exercise to your routine per the instructions in Chapter 7, even if it's a short walk after meals. Also, make sure your meter is calibrated (refer to manufacturer instructions) and your blood sugar strips are not expired.

Keep a detailed Food & Blood Sugar Log so you can track trends in blood sugar levels based on these changes. Also, if you are sick or under a lot of stress, your blood sugar may temporarily spike, but will return to normal soon after. That's why tracking blood sugar trends is so helpful!

Even if your blood sugar levels don't come all the way down to normal, you're not necessarily doing anything wrong! It's always a bit of an experiment. Nonetheless, you've provided your baby with more nourishing food and healthy movement. None of that effort was wasted. I know it's frustrating, but every woman's metabolism is different and sometimes you'll need a little help from medicine or insulin to fully bring your blood sugar down to normal. Taking medication is not "giving up" or "failing". Rather, it's the healthiest thing you can do for your baby in this instance. Chapter 8 gives you in-depth information on the blood sugar medications commonly used during pregnancy. Talk to your medical provider about your options.

If you are already taking insulin/medication, talk to your medical provider about adjusting your dose, timing, or routine. It's not uncommon to need higher doses of blood sugar medicine later in pregnancy.

I feel hungry all the time! What can I eat that won't spike my blood sugar?

Remember, as your baby grows, you'll get hungry - and for good reason! Some women go through spurts where they feel like no matter how much they eat, they're still hungry. As long as you're choosing nutrient-dense foods and limiting high-carbohydrate and refined foods, you're fine! Your baby goes through the most rapid period of growth from weeks 22 to term, so don't be surprised if you're hungrier and gaining weight quicker during the second half of pregnancy. Check out the healthy snacks list included in Chapter 4 for some inspiration. Be sure to include some protein and fat with your snacks to keep you satiated without spiking your blood sugar (and of course, don't forget to eat your veggies!). Listen to your body and never let yourself get too hungry.

I'm having a hard time giving up pasta, bread, and carbohydrates. What are some alternatives?

You don't necessarily have to omit these foods entirely, but you may need to reduce them. It takes time to adjust to a new way of eating. When it comes to pasta, you can start by adding extra vegetables (chopped broccoli or spinach to the tomato sauce) and yummy proteins (like meatballs and shredded cheese) to your pasta dishes to help reduce your consumption of pasta without feeling deprived. Some women also make noodles out of zucchini using a vegetable peeler or a "spiralizer" (a gadget specifically designed to make noodles out of vegetables). A good compromise is to make a 50:50 mix of regular spaghetti and zucchini noodles. Spaghetti squash is also a lower-carb noodle replacement.

Bread is a tough one to give up. You can try eating open-faced sandwiches (1 slice of bread) or switch over to lettuce wraps.

114

Many sandwich fillings are delicious on top of a salad.

In place of rice, you can make "riced" cauliflower by grating raw cauliflower (or pulsing in the food processor) and then baking on a sheet pan in a 425 degree oven for 15 minutes. Cauliflower can also be cooked and mashed just like potatoes. Get creative and have fun experimenting in the kitchen! These are skills you'll use for the rest of your life.

I'm craving sweets. Are there any GD-friendly desserts?

If you recently began changing your diet, know that your sugar cravings will decrease over time. That being said, I believe we should all indulge a little bit, and do so in a way that minimizes blood sugar spikes. One half cup of fresh fruit with a heaping dollop of freshly whipped cream (flavored with vanilla extract and perhaps a little stevia) is a great option. Or try 1-2 ounces of dark chocolate (75% cocoa or more) with a small handful of nuts. Homemade custard, made primarily with a base of egg yolks and heavy cream, is another indulgent, yet nutritious option. Like any carbohydrates, matching your sweets with a source of fat or protein will satisfy with less impact on your blood sugar.

Since I changed my diet, I've lost a little weight. Is that normal?

Most women lose a few pounds when they reduce carbohydrates and eliminate junk foods, partly due to decreased inflammation and fluid accumulation when blood sugar and insulin levels drop. So, minor weight loss is normal in the first few weeks on a gestational diabetes diet. Chances are your weight will stabilize after that point. Discuss your weight gain goals with your doctor to be sure you're on target. Eating enough fat and protein while minimizing carbohydrates does a marvelous job of normalizing hunger and fullness cues in your body, so you may notice you have fewer cravings or urges to overeat. That's a *good* thing!

I have nausea and vomiting. What can I do?

It's tough, isn't it? You want to do everything to nourish your baby, and yet your body is rejecting food. Hang in there and give a couple of these options a whirl. Start by tracking your major triggers. Is it strong odors? Time of day? Certain foods? Movement? Getting too hungry? Overeating? Eating too fast?

Most women benefit from smaller, more frequent snacks in place of large meals when nausea is at its worst. This helps prevent you from getting too hungry or too full, both common nausea triggers. You might also try supplementing with vitamin B6 or munching on vitamin B6-rich foods, like avocado, banana (careful with your portion size), pistachios, and sunflower seeds. Magnesium has also been shown to lessen nausea and morning sickness. You can either take a supplement or do a relaxing foot bath with epsom salt to boost your levels. Also refer to Chapter 6 for a list of magnesium-rich foods. Lastly, try ginger! Ginger has been used for centuries to reduce nausea.

Carbohydrates tend to be the easiest-to-digest foods, so if you're having trouble stomaching any food, opt for things like fruit, cooked sweet potatoes, or rice. Just be aware that sharp blood sugar fluctuations are another nausea trigger. So once you can tolerate a little carbohydrates, try to follow with a small portion of protein or fat-containing foods to stabilize your blood sugar. It's not a perfect science, but it's worth a try.

If you do happen to throw up, be sure to replenish lost fluids and electrolytes with homemade broth, diluted juice, coconut water, and anything salty. If you are unable to keep *anything* down (food or fluids), call your provider, as dehydration can be dangerous.

I'm not hungry for snacks. Should I eat them anyways?

In short, no. You should always listen to your body, which means eating when you're hungry and stopping when you're full, but not stuffed. So, if you're a person who doesn't get hungry between meals, don't eat a snack just because I say so. However, if you're noticing your blood sugar is high after meals or you have low energy between meals, you might benefit from eating smaller portions at meals and including snacks throughout the day. Also, many women notice improved fasting blood sugar when they include a bedtime snack. By your third trimester, when your stomach is being compressed from the baby, you might need snacks just to consume enough energy and nutrients (and avoid heartburn!). If you take insulin or glyburide, you'll likely require snacks to prevent low blood sugar between meals.

Summary

As you can see, there are many possible causes and solutions to these complaints. Your job is to pay attention, remain curious, and experiment with what works best for you. And remember, you *can* figure this out!

For more strategies on managing your gestational diabetes, including GD-friendly recipes, real food tips for pregnancy, and prenatal exercise, visit **www.RealFoodforGD.com**.

Erin's Story

When I got pregnant, gestational diabetes was the furthest thing from my mind. When I had my glucose tolerance test, I was shocked it came out positive. I have a history of polycystic ovarian syndrome (PCOS) and was on metformin already, but I was at a healthy weight and I got pregnant easily. I really didn't think I was at risk. It was actually very upsetting because I was forced to leave my midwife. That meant changing my prenatal care plan and being followed by a diabetes team.

I was recommended to eat 175g of carbohydrates and stay on my metformin (which was for my PCOS). Personally, I found 175g of carbohydrates to be way too high for me. Instead, I ate 10-15 g of carbohydrates at breakfast, 15-25g at lunch and dinner, lower carbohydrates snacks during the day, and 20g at my bedtime snack. By eating that way my post-meal blood sugar was pretty good, but my fasting blood sugar remained borderline high.

I experimented a lot with trying to lower my fasting blood sugar. Oddly enough, eating some ice cream before bed helped drop my fasting blood sugar a little. But as the weeks went on it became clear I needed insulin. So at around 20 weeks, I was started on NPH insulin at night. That was able to bring my fasting blood sugar to normal levels.

Eventually my post-meal numbers started creeping up, so the doctors added insulin with my meals. But what was scary about this is that I had a few serious hypoglycemia episodes (blood sugar in the 40s). Unfortunately, my diabetes team didn't identify this pattern until very late in my pregnancy. It turns out that when I would take the insulin with my meals, my blood sugar would be fine one hour later (when I checked my post-meal blood sugar). But two hours after the meal, my blood sugar would drop too low. Frankly, it was frustrating, frightening, and I just felt there wasn't enough guidance.

Aside from all of this, I was able to keep my blood sugar close to normal the majority of the time. I stayed active my whole pregnancy, running until 35 weeks. And thankfully, my baby was born at a normal weight with no complications.

Postpartum, my fasting blood sugars were over 100, showing that I was still prediabetic (despite exclusively breastfeeding). I continued to test my blood sugar and my fasting blood sugar only dropped to normal levels (in the 80s) when I lowered my carbohydrate levels.

Next pregnancy, I will choose to go lower carbohydrate, so I don't have to take insulin (or at least not as much) and don't have hypoglycemia. I realize I'll likely still need insulin at night, and I may even need some at meals, but I'd rather be proactive and change what I eat so I can take smaller doses.

The good thing about gestational diabetes is that I now realize I was probably always prediabetic, so I know what to watch. I know how food impacts my blood sugar and I can choose to eat in a way to keep my blood sugar normal, so I don't end up with type 2 diabetes and being insulin dependent by the time I'm in my 40s.

Chapter 10

Postpartum Strategies to Keep You and Baby Healthy

Once your baby is born, your work has just begun. Some people refer to this as the "fourth trimester," as just like pregnancy, caring for a newborn can be a bit of a roller coaster. It's certainly a learning process, especially if this is your first baby!

You may have been told that gestational diabetes is something you only need to worry about during pregnancy and that it goes away once your baby is born. That's partially true. Without the influence of placental hormones, your blood sugar will likely decrease after you give birth, but we now know women who have had gestational diabetes have at least a 50% chance of developing type 2 diabetes by the time their baby turns five.

Remember, gestational diabetes is often the first warning sign that your body has difficulty regulating your blood sugar (insulin resistance), and it affects different women to varying degrees. Luckily, there is a lot you can do to reduce your chances of developing type 2 diabetes and that's the purpose for this chapter. You did everything within your power to have a healthy pregnancy, so let's continue on that path and keep YOU healthy long term!

Breastfeeding

One of the best ways to ensure you and your baby stay healthy is to breastfeed. You've probably already heard about all the usual benefits for the baby, so let's focus on the benefits to your health for a change.

Breastfeeding helps to lower your blood sugar and insulin levels. Here's why: The mammary glands use glucose to synthesize lactose, thereby lowering serum blood sugar (without insulin). Plus, insulin sensitivity increases during lactation due to hormonal changes, namely increased prolactin levels and decreased cortisol and estrogen. Breastfeeding also has a direct impact on the pancreas. In fact, women who had gestational diabetes have improved beta cell function (the cells in your pancreas that make insulin) after only 3 months of breastfeeding.[98] But don't stop at 3 months! The longer you breastfeed, the lower your chances of developing type 2 diabetes later in life.[99] For every year a woman breastfeeds, her chance of developing type 2 diabetes drops by 14%. On the flipside, women who had gestational diabetes who choose not to breastfeed, have a 50% increased risk of developing type 2 diabetes.[100]

Breastfeeding also helps you lose the weight gained during pregnancy, which by itself has many healthy benefits. Women who exclusively breastfeed burn an average of 500 additional calories per day, which is equivalent to the energy expended in a 2-hour walk.

As Dr. Siri Kjos says, "It's like having a gym on your chest!"

Of course, the benefits extend to your infant as well. Aside from the immune, cognitive, and digestive benefits, breastfeeding can help reduce the chance that your baby will become overweight or develop diabetes in his or her lifetime. Researchers believe breastfeeding could offset some of the negative effects of being exposed to high blood sugar levels during gestation. In one study, infants of moms with gestational diabetes who were breastfed for more than 6 months had significantly lower adiposity (body fat) at 6-13 years of age compared to those who were breastfed for less than 6 months.[101]

Since research has shown that prenatal nutrition and early exposure to breastfeeding can impact the likelihood that offspring will develop diabetes and obesity, sometimes referred to as a transgenerational cycle, your choice to breastfeed could have lasting effects on your children and even your grandchildren. How amazing is that?

Postpartum Nutrition

What you eat after your baby is born is just as important as what you ate during pregnancy. In general, you can continue your nutrient-dense prenatal diet with a few modifications.

If you are breastfeeding, you will likely be pretty hungry! That's because your body can expend up to 500 extra calories a day producing milk (200 more calories compared to the energy you needed while pregnant)." For many moms, the challenge is finding the time to prepare food and eat while juggling a newborn. Consider cooking meals in advance and having healthy, easy-to-grab snacks handy. In addition to higher energy needs, your body requires more fluids while breastfeeding, so choose plenty of unsweetened beverages to stay hydrated. A good rule of thumb is to have 8oz of fluids and a small snack (if you're hungry) with each feeding.

While breast milk is healthy no matter what you eat, remember that you can produce higher quality and more nutritious breast milk if you're eating well. Stick to real foods with clean ingredient labels (no artificial flavors, food dyes, trans fats, corn syrup, etc) and be sure to consume enough non-starchy vegetables, fat, and protein to stay satiated. Long term, a diet moderately low in carbohydrates, as outlined in Chapters 3 and 4 is ideal.

Vitamins and Nutrients of Concern

It's wise to continue your prenatal vitamin and vitamin D supplement even after birth, at least while you're breastfeeding. Sadly, most breast milk is low in vitamin D, a reflection of poor vitamin D status in the mother. Breast milk, on average, contains only 10 to 80 IUs of vitamin D per liter while formula is standardized to contain 400 IU/liter.[102] That explains why exclusively breastfed infants have higher rates of rickets compared to formula-fed infants. The answer is not to formula-feed your infant, but to be vigilant about your vitamin D levels and your vitamin D supplements. A large randomized controlled trial showed that breastfeeding moms supplemented with 4000 IU/day had higher vitamin D levels, breast milk richer in vitamin D, and infants with better vitamin D status at 4 months compared to moms given half that dose.[103] In addition, all infants should receive 400 IU of vitamin D per day in supplemental form according to the American Academy of Pediatrics.

If you were taking fish oil or DHA supplements while pregnant, continue taking those while breastfeeding. Early exposure to these omega-3 fatty acids can impact cognitive and eye development *for life*. If you do not take those supplements, be sure to consume fatty fish a few times per week, such as wild salmon, sardines or herring.

Choline needs increase during breastfeeding compared to pregnancy levels. That's because choline is crucial for brain development and readily transferred through breastmilk.[104] Breastfeeding women require 550mg of choline at minimum per day: the amount found in approximately 4 egg yolks. You may also consider obtaining choline from eating the liver of pasture-raised animals, the richest known dietary source of choline (and many other vitamins). Only 3 ounces of beef liver provides a whopping 420mg of choline; 3 ounces of chicken liver has 290mg. Liver is also extremely rich in iron, another nutrient moms and babies tend to be deficient in.

Weight Loss

After baby is born, most women are eager to lose the weight they gained during pregnancy. Your body has done something miraculous and you have this wonderful baby in your arms; however, taking care of yourself is just as important as caring for your baby. Without good health, you can't be the best mother possible. And you certainly don't want to develop type

2 diabetes in the next decade.

So while I don't recommend you focus too much on the numbers on the scale, I do suggest you take a look at where you are currently and what weight would be healthy and comfortable for you to maintain. It's not about vanity, it's about health.

First, look at your prepregnancy weight.

Were you underweight, normal weight, overweight, or obese before becoming pregnant?
How much weight did you gain during the pregnancy?
What's a realistic and healthy weight for you to maintain?

Ideally, women should lose the weight gained during pregnancy within six months of delivery. Some women are able to do this more rapidly and sometimes it takes longer. The rate at which you lose weight will depend on your prepregnancy weight and how much weight you gained during the pregnancy, but beware that restrictive eating while breastfeeding can reduce your milk supply. Aim to lose 1-2 pounds per week unless you were very overweight preconception or you exceeded your doctor's prenatal weight gain recommendations. (And remember, if you gained 25-35 pounds during your pregnancy, typically half that weight is lost at delivery and a few more pounds come off during the next few days as swelling subsides).

No matter what, be sure you eat consistently and choose nutrient-dense foods (as described in previous chapters), so you're losing weight healthfully. The ultimate goal is that you'll attain a healthy weight postpartum not only for your own health, but for the health of your future children, should you choose to have more.

Women who lose just 7-10% of their body weight have a 50% reduced risk of developing type 2 diabetes.[105] That means if you weigh 175 pounds, you only need to lose 12-18 pounds to fully *halve* your risk of diabetes. Pretty amazing!

Exercise

Aside from good nutrition, exercise can help you stay healthy and lose the weight gained during pregnancy. Typically, you should wait 6 weeks to resume your usual exercise regimen unless you have doctor's approval to start sooner. Women who've had C-sections or complicated deliveries may need longer to heal. Listen to your body and respect what it has to say.

Start slow when you begin exercising. Consider low-impact exercises, such as walking, Pilates, and gentle yoga. The pelvic floor and abdominal exercises I cover in Chapter 7 are great places to start. Many women have pelvic floor issues following birth and some countries, such as France and Japan, refer *all* postpartum moms to specialized women's physical therapy. Don't hesitate to request a referral from your doctor if you're having pain or discomfort with exercise or intercourse.

Testing for Diabetes Postpartum

For most women, blood sugars return to normal after delivery. But for some women, blood sugar issues can persist. Other times, blood sugars may temporarily return to normal, particularly if you're breastfeeding, and then become problematic in the first few years after delivery. This is why it's crucial to follow up with your doctor periodically and get tested for diabetes.

A systematic review and meta-analysis of over 650,000 women found that women with gestational diabetes are *seven times* more likely to develop type 2 diabetes than women with no blood sugar issues during pregnancy.[106] Women who have high fasting blood sugar during pregnancy have a higher risk of developing type 2 diabetes compared to women with high post-meal blood sugars. The statistics are staggering and you've had an early warning sign, but you can take control of your health and steer this ship in another direction by following the advice in this book.

126

Your doctor should test your blood sugar between 6-12 weeks postpartum and again around your child's first birthday. Every doctor screens differently. They may choose to test your fasting blood sugar, random glucose check, perform an oral glucose tolerance test, or measure hemoglobin A1c.

If your numbers are abnormal, your doctor should check again 1 year later, as many women "convert" to type 2 diabetes if they don't make changes to their diet and exercise habits. If your numbers at the one-year screening come back normal, your doctor should repeat screening at minimum every 3 years (some continue to check annually).

Future Pregnancies

Since you developed gestational diabetes with this pregnancy, chances are you'll have gestational diabetes with future pregnancies. The recurrence rate of GD varies from 30% to 84%.[107] You may be able to offset that risk by changing your lifestyle and achieving a healthy weight before conceiving again. There's always the variable impact of placental hormones on insulin resistance, which may remain somewhat out of our control.

A good way to estimate your risk of developing gestational diabetes is to have your hemoglobin A1c measured early in pregnancy. This test measures your average blood sugar over 3 months. When this number is greater than 5.7% (the cutoff for prediabetes), progressive doctors will treat you as having gestational diabetes. But if your doctor is not so keen and decides to wait until 24-28 weeks to perform a glucose tolerance test, know this: A first trimester A1c of 5.9% or greater accurately predicts gestational diabetes 98.4% of the time.[108]

In my eyes, you're better off knowing early and eating in a way that promotes normal blood sugar and normal weight gain than waiting until half of your pregnancy has passed. The nutrition advice given in this book is healthy for any pregnant woman, with or without gestational diabetes, so you can always return to this pattern of eating with your next pregnancy. (Ideally, you'll eat this way for the rest of your life!)

One study found that the combination of not smoking, exercising 150 minutes or more per week, and healthy eating reduced the risk of gestational diabetes by 41%.[109] Another study found that women who regularly exercised during the year prior to conception and through 20 weeks gestation had a 49-78% reduced risk of gestational diabetes.[110] While these particular studies were not looking specifically at women with a previous diagnosis of gestational diabetes, it does reinforce the power we have over our health outcomes.

Aside from your preconception weight, diet, and exercise levels, some other factors may prevent gestational diabetes. This includes supplementation with probiotics and maintaining normal vitamin D levels. One study found that supplementing women with probiotics starting in the first trimester reduced the risk of gestational diabetes by 20%.[111] This is a very new area of research, but one that merits attention. Deficiency in vitamin D is associated with insulin resistance and increases the risk of developing gestational diabetes. Refer to chapter 6 for more information about vitamin D and probiotics.

Summary

My hope is that you'll use this information to be proactive about your health. Think of getting diagnosed with gestational diabetes as the "check engine" light coming on in your car. You know that your blood sugar is always something you need to be aware of, but as long as you're on top of maintenance (real food, movement, etc.), you'll cruise along just fine.

You've been lucky enough to understand and practice eating in a way that keeps your blood sugar normal throughout this pregnancy, so I have no doubt you'll be able to continue. It's not fate or destiny that you'll develop type 2 diabetes later in life. That, my friend, you have some control over. Cheers to your healthy baby and a lifetime of good health!

Wendy's Story

In my first pregnancy, I started at a normal weight and followed the standard nutrition advice from my doctor, which was a low fat diet, lots of fruit, and what I believed to be healthy. I ended up putting on about 45 pounds and almost failed my glucose tolerance test. After this pregnancy, I tried to stick with these same nutrition recommendations to lose the weight I had gained during the pregnancy. I was only able to drop *some* of the weight by exercising many hours a day. It was pure torture. Years later, I had gained back all the weight and then some.

At this point, we were having trouble trying to conceive when I came across the low carb diet to help boost fertility and potentially fix the other health issues I was dealing with. Just by cutting back on carbohydrates a little, I lost 20 pounds easily and felt dramatically better - my energy was back, my headaches went away, and food finally didn't seem like a struggle.

By the time I got pregnant the second time, I had been eating a low carbohydrate diet for about 6 months (with gradual weight loss), however I was still 100 pounds overweight. While I felt great and I knew this diet had helped me lose weight, all the research I found online said that a low carbohydrate diet could be dangerous in pregnancy. It scared me out of my mind.

With a lot of reading, I ended up deciding to keep my carbohydrates to 50-100g of carbs per day (15-20g carbs per meal) and focused on whole foods. I ended up gaining exactly 20 pounds by the time I delivered, which was what my doctor recommended, passed the glucose tolerance test (despite being 10 years older, and heavier than my first pregnancy), and never struggled with the fatigue that I had the first time around. My low carb baby had a higher Apgar score at birth and was also more alert than my first. I had been so afraid of harming my baby's development by eating low carb, but it just goes to show this was definitely not the case.

The difference between my two pregnancies was like night and day. With my second pregnancy I didn't have any issues with low energy, excessive weight gain, or postpartum depression. Plus within 2 months postpartum after my low carb pregnancy, I was actually below my preconception weight! I hope more moms will consider a low carb diet during their pregnancy.

Chapter 11

Questioning the Conventional Dietary Approach to Gestational Diabetes

The purpose of this chapter is to provide evidence and reassurance that the dietary recommendations I present in this book are safe, efficacious, and actually *ideal* for a healthy pregnancy. You'll notice that I have chosen to include this information at the end of this book. In my opinion, the dietary management of gestational diabetes is actually quite simple; this section is fairly complex.

I've made a choice to keep this book as straightforward as possible, but the following research-heavy section is necessary for moms (or even healthcare practitioners) who, like me, believe that a lower carbohydrate diet is safe for pregnancy and are up against scrutiny from others for choosing this path.

When Conventional Diet Therapy Fails

When I first started working as a prenatal nutritionist, I dutifully followed the standard nutrition guidelines for gestational diabetes: 175g of carbohydrates minimum for women in their second and third trimester of pregnancy. Only there was one problem: my patients' blood sugar numbers were *not* improving.

Unless they were previously consuming a very-high-carbohydrate diet (which, of course, I did also see), this level of carbohydrates wasn't low enough to bring their blood sugar down to normal. Sometimes their blood sugar got *worse* when they implemented the dietary changes I suggested, much to our mutual disappointment. Sooner or later, they needed the help of insulin or medication. Actually, quite a high percentage needed the help of medicine. And that just seemed wrong to me.

Sadly, it's accepted that at least 40% of women will "fail diet therapy".[112] But I have to wonder - does that mean these women failed, or does it mean our dietary recommendations *failed them*? Why would we recommend a diet that perpetuated the use of medication and insulin if we had another option?

My initial instinct was to suggest a diet lower in carbohydrates. After all, gestational diabetes is defined as *carbohydrate intolerance*. And we already know that a low-glycemic index diet (that includes slowly digested, unrefined carbohydrates) can reduce the need for insulin by 50% in women with gestational diabetes.[113] I figured that a diet lower in *total* carbohydrates could reduce the need for insulin even more and ease the strain on an already overworked pancreas, just as does for people with type 2 diabetes.

But, the argument against decreasing *total* carbohydrates during pregnancy was clear: a low-carbohydrate diet might induce ketosis. Ketosis is essentially another word for "fat burning". When your diet is limited in carbohydrates, your body will preferentially burn fat for fuel instead of carbohydrates. When in "fat burning mode", your body releases compounds called ketones. From all the training I had received, I was told that ketones would be harmful to a growing fetus and therefore women should consume enough carbohydrates to stay out of ketosis.

At the same time, I was hearing from my patients that eating 45 grams (or more) of carbohydrates at meals was just too much. They were too full, their blood sugar was too high, they struggled with sugar cravings, and they were gaining too much weight despite diligently following my advice. It just went against common sense to force upon them food that they were not hungry for, particularly more carbohydrates, when their blood sugar was already elevated.

Thus began my quest to uncover how the carbohydrate recommendations for pregnant women were formulated. Plus, I wanted to understand for myself if ketones were really a problem (or not) for a developing baby.

Why Standard Carbohydrate Recommendations Are Wrong

What I uncovered shocked me. There was absolutely no solid data to support the magical 175g of carbohydrates per day that dietitians, like myself, had militantly followed.

Here's how that number was decided upon:

You start with the Estimated Average Requirement for non-pregnant women of 100g of carbohydrates per day. Then add 35g, to account for the increased energy demand of pregnancy (approximately 300 calories, divided by the recommended percentage of dietary carbohydrates of at least 45%, divided by 4 calories per gram of carbohydrate). Finally, you add 33g, which is the amount of glucose estimated to be required by the fetal brain per day. Those numbers taken together, plus a little buffer (very scientific, right?), give us 175g per day.

Now this all sounds reasonable, assuming the evidence behind the dietary guidelines is infallible. But in fact, when you read the fine print within the 1,357-page document defending the carbohydrate levels indicated, you find this:

"The lower limit of dietary carbohydrate compatible with life apparently is zero, provided that adequate amounts of protein and fat are consumed."[114]

That alone negates the Estimated Average Requirements of 100g per day, leaving us with 75g of carbohydrate per day, which is by most definitions a moderately low-carbohydrate diet.

Of course, many people subsist just fine on a low-carbohydrate diet, including traditional cultures (Masai, Inuit, Australian Aboriginals, Alaska and Greenland Natives) who follow this diet throughout their lifetime, presumably also during pregnancy. That's because our bodies have the ability to produce much of the glucose we need from fat and protein.

"In the absence of dietary carbohydrate, de novo synthesis of glucose requires amino acids derived from the hydrolysis of endogenous or dietary protein or glycerol derived from fat. Therefore, the marginal amount of carbohydrate required in the diet in an energy-balanced state is conditional and dependent upon the remaining composition of the diet."[114]

When our bodies are in this state of nutritional ketosis described above, circulating glucose and insulin concentrations naturally drop by 20-50%.[114] This would seem advantageous to a pregnancy complicated by gestational diabetes. And indeed, normal pregnancies actually favor a state of ketosis.

"As part of the adaptation to pregnancy, there is a decrease in maternal blood glucose concentration, a development of insulin resistance, and a tendency to develop ketosis."[114]

This again brought up the question of how safe it is for a mother to be in ketosis while pregnant. My intention was not necessarily to provide a ketogenic diet to my patients, but to fully understand the risks of occasionally dipping into ketosis from eating a diet moderately low in carbohydrates.

Why, if ketosis was harmful, would pregnancy perpetuate this metabolic state?

Nutritional Ketosis, Starvation Ketosis, and Diabetic Ketoacidosis

Before I go any further, I have to define the different types of ketosis because they are often not differentiated. I believe this is the primary reason ketosis is so feared during pregnancy.

Nutritional ketosis refers to a state where the body is burning primarily fat for fuel because the diet is limited in carbohydrates, but not energy (adequate calories from fat and protein). In nutritional ketosis, blood sugar levels are normal. Nutritional ketosis is the state that a pregnant woman might experience if she eats a lower carbohydrate diet.

Starvation ketosis happens when your body is burning primarily stored body fat for fuel because the person is eating inadequate calories from all sources.

Finally, *diabetic ketoacidosis* (DKA) is a state that *only* occurs in people with type 1 diabetes or insulin-dependent type 2 diabetes, when they have inadequate insulin to allow their body to use glucose. This is classically due to skipping insulin shots, incorrectly dosing insulin, or taking inadequate insulin to cover unexpected elevations in blood sugar. Unlike nutritional ketosis or starvation ketosis, DKA is accompanied by unnaturally high levels of ketones from complete insulin deprivation and blood sugar levels at least 3 times higher than normal, which profoundly *and dangerously* alters the acid-base balance in the body. The blood sugar levels seen with DKA are themselves teratogenic (can cause birth defects), so this state should obviously be avoided by pregnant women. Some studies have suggested the metabolic effects of diabetic ketoacidosis may harm fetal neuropsychomotor development.[115]

Unfortunately, many medical providers incorrectly associate nutritional ketosis (or just the word "ketosis") with diabetic ketoacidosis, a known medical emergency, when in fact the type of ketosis a pregnant woman with gestational diabetes is most likely to encounter, provided she's eating adequate calories, is mild nutritional ketosis.

Low-Level Ketosis Is Common in Pregnancy

If mild ketosis was truly harmful in pregnancy, women who experienced morning sickness, hyperemesis gravidarum, severe food aversions, or even those who skip breakfast wouldn't be able to carry a healthy child to term. Also, any traditional cultures that subsisted on a low-carbohydrate diet would also not have been able to successfully reproduce.

Of course, unless a woman has gestational diabetes or preexisting diabetes, measuring for ketones is not standard practice, so it's hard to know for sure how many pregnant women experience ketosis. Yet studies have shown that even healthy, non-diabetic pregnant women will have marked elevation in ketones after a 12-18 hour fast, which is akin to eating dinner at 8pm and having breakfast at 8am (or skipping breakfast entirely).[116] Compared to non-pregnant women, blood ketone concentrations are about 3-fold higher in healthy pregnant women after an overnight fast.[117] Knowing this, I would expect that *every* pregnant woman experiences ketosis at some point during her pregnancy.

In late pregnancy, ketosis is even more likely as maternal metabolism shifts to favor catabolism, or in other words, the breaking down of maternal fat stores to supply the fetus with increased levels of nutrients.[118] Naturally, this results in ketosis, particularly between meals and overnight.

"Under fasting conditions, fatty acids are converted into ketone bodies throughout the beta-oxidation pathway, and these compounds easily cross the placental barrier and are metabolized by the fetus."[118]

So how do you know if you are in ketosis? And how do you know if you're at a safe level?

Urine Ketones vs. Blood Ketones

In some medical practices, women with gestational diabetes are screened for ketones at each visit and some are taught to measure ketones at home. Ketones are typically measured from urine with a simple dipstick.

But, this practice is perplexing, given that urinary ketones do not accurately reflect blood ketone levels, particularly during pregnancy. One study of 146 pregnant women (diabetic and non-diabetic) on low-calorie diets (1000-1800 kcal/day) had urinary and blood ketones measured regularly during their second and third trimesters. In 120 instances (11% of the total tests), urinary ketones were detected, but *not once* were plasma ketones positive.

In fact, urinary ketones may increase 50 to 100-fold while blood ketones will only rise 2-fold and remain below ketonemic levels (defined as levels at or above 1mmol/L).[119] That means a woman can test for "large" urinary ketones, sending healthcare providers in a tizzy, even when blood ketones are at trace and non-harmful levels.

In fact, during this study, the highest levels of blood ketones detected was 0.34mmol/L. True diabetic ketoacidosis typically appears at blood ketone levels of 10-20mmol/L, at least 30-fold higher than the *highest* level recorded throughout this study. That means that even women subjected to very-low-calorie diets (which, in this case, were also low in carbohydrates) didn't experience harmful levels of ketones in their blood.

It's unknown whether the damaging effects of diabetic ketoacidosis are due to the unnaturally high ketone levels, high blood glucose levels, or improper acid-base balance (it's likely all three), but just for an example, if we assume that the acid-base balance is to blame, note that a ketone level of at least 5mmol/L is needed to alter acid-base balance.[120] This is still 15-fold higher than the *highest* level recorded in this study.

No study since this one, as far as I'm aware, has tracked urine *and* blood ketone levels throughout pregnancy. And furthermore, few studies have tested such a low-calorie diet in pregnancy, which by default, is ketogenic and far more restricted in calories than I would ever deem adequate for pregnancy.

This knowledge has led many providers to abandon urine ketone testing entirely. The California Diabetes and Pregnancy Program only suggests measuring urinary ketones in women with preexisting diabetes (type 1 and type 2 diabetes), particularly those taking insulin. Even then, testing positive for urinary ketones is only a red flag if a woman *also* has hyperglycemia, which could indicate diabetic ketoacidosis. But ketonuria is *not* diagnostic of diabetic ketoacidosis alone and must be confirmed through blood ketone tests. As outlined in the California Diabetes and Pregnancy Program *Guidelines For Care*:

"Diagnosis of diabetic ketoacidosis (DKA) is not made on the basis of ketonuria but on the basis of hyperglycemia, ketonemia and low bicarbonate level which is a medical emergency."

Based on my clinical experience and the scientific literature, when it comes to gestational diabetes, routine ketone testing should be abandoned.

Will Ketones Hurt the Baby?

If you've done any reading on low-carbohydrate diets during pregnancy, you've been warned that ketones hurt the baby, but that's not the full story. Whether or not ketones are problematic depends on the type of ketosis and the level of ketones in the bloodstream. As I already outlined, diabetic ketoacidosis is *never* safe due to unnaturally high levels of glucose, ketones, and imbalanced blood pH.

Starvation ketosis is also not ideal because inadequate food deprives the mother of more than just glucose. Yes, starvation will induce ketosis, but it also means a mother is depleted of essential fatty acids, amino acids, vitamins, minerals, micronutrients, and antioxidants (and other compounds found in real food we have yet to discover). So we can't rely on starvation studies to prove that *ketosis* is harmful. You cannot separate the effects of ketosis from the effects of complete nutrient deprivation.

In fact, we know maternal calorie deprivation "profoundly alters the levels of amino acids in amniotic fluid" and promotes hypoglycemia.[121] Under no circumstances would it make sense for starvation to be a good thing for a mother and growing fetus, but a diet that provides adequate calories and low amounts of carbohydrates is *not* starvation. Plus, a low-carbohydrate diet, in the absence of medication or insulin, actually protects against hypoglycemia.[122]

Nutritional ketosis -- where a mom is taking in adequate calories, protein, fat, vitamins, minerals, and limited amounts of carbohydrates -- would be unlikely to be problematic. Here's why.

When ketones are suggested as being harmful in fetal development, people reference either diabetic ketoacidosis or a single study from 1969. This study suggested that maternal urinary ketones were associated with lower IQ in young children.[123] However, this study is deeply flawed, as it's based on reports from hospital nurses checking a single urine ketone test from women the day of delivery. Blood ketones were not checked, which, as outlined above, are the only reliable way to ascertain ketone levels.

As one researcher put it, "urine ketone levels bear little relation to blood levels once the acetoacetate values [a type of ketone] reach values as low as 0.1 mmol/L, which is 100 times less than is needed to depress cerebral oxygen utilization."[119]

This study reassures us that positive urinary ketone tests during pregnancy do not indicate harmful blood ketone levels: "Neonates born to diabetic mothers with ketonuria had no fetal distress or asphyxia neonatorum [when a baby fails to breathe normally at birth]. The lowest Apgar score at 5 min was 8; 80% of neonates had a score of 10. Hence, positive Ketostix tests in urine samples do not indicate toxic levels in the blood."[119] In fact, in this study, women who tested positive for ketones had infants with slightly *higher* Apgar scores.

Rat studies confirm that ketones present at physiological levels (those seen with low carbohydrate diets) do *not* cause developmental malformations.[124]

Remember, the only way ketones reach toxic levels is diabetic ketoacidosis.[125] Low levels of ketones are not a concern, and surprisingly, may provide benefits.

Ketones May Be Good for Baby

Despite all the medical warnings about ketones, it turns out the fetal brain actually gets approximately 30% of its energy from ketones.[114]

"Since ketone bodies can be used by the brain (including fetal brain) as natural fuel, and there is evidence that the synthesis of essential cerebral lipids occurs from these substances, it is inconceivable that the blood levels reached during calorie-restricted diets could cause harm."[119]

Did you catch that? Ketones are actually used by the growing fetus to synthesize *essential cerebral lipids*! Perhaps this is why pregnancy naturally favors low-level ketosis; to help, not hinder, fetal brain development. It makes sense, then, that moms who test positive for urinary ketones during pregnancy (again, not diabetic ketoacidosis, but nutritional ketosis) give birth to perfectly healthy infants. The low level of ketones in moms who eat a low-carbohydrate diet may actually be beneficial!

Research into ketone metabolism in the growing fetus and infants has shown that at least 13% of the total cerebral oxygen consumption at 2 and 4 weeks of neonatal life comes from ketones.[126]

During an infant's first few days of life, ketones account for 25% of their energy needs.[127] This explains why babies are born with so much brown fat. This serves as the primary fuel source for exclusively-breastfed infants for the first 3 days after delivery until a mother's lactose-rich breast milk comes in.

And get this: Ketones are so important for fetal development, that researchers believe the fetus manufactures its own ketones. Umbilical venous blood samples (fetal blood supply) indicate significantly higher ketone concentrations compared to maternal levels in healthy pregnant women in their second and third trimesters.[128]

So although the fetus requires glucose for growth, it also requires ketones. Either fuel provided in excess is harmful to the developing fetus, but as long as a mom is consuming enough calories and maintaining normal blood sugar levels, the baby will get just the right mix.

When Ketosis May Be Favorable for Mom

Ketosis may actually be beneficial for moms as well. A high percentage of women with gestational diabetes are overweight at conception or have exceeded their weight gain goals established by their doctor. These women have increased fat stores that can supply energy for the growing fetus and do not necessarily benefit from continued weight gain. Some studies actually found no weight gain or modest weight *loss* during pregnancy can improve outcomes in obese women.[129]

Suggesting the standard high-carbohydrate diet purely to keep women out of ketosis results in hyperglycemia and the need for medication, usually insulin, which often results in excess weight gain. With weight gain comes a worsening of peripheral insulin resistance, which results in higher blood sugar and the need for ever increasing doses of insulin and medication. It's a vicious cycle. Plus, the majority of macrosomic babies are born to mothers with excessive weight gain and prepregnancy obesity, *not* gestational diabetes.[130]

In fact, women who gain an excessive amount of weight during pregnancy have triple the risk of giving birth to a macrosomic baby and a 1.5 times higher risk of their baby being born with hypoglycemia and jaundice.[131]   Therefore, focusing only on glycemic control and the avoidance of urinary ketones at the expense of weight gain goals is counterproductive.

Consuming a carbohydrate-restricted diet favors moderate weight gain (or even weight loss in some women), normal blood sugars, and in some, will happen to result in nutritional ketosis. For overweight women, achieving the strict weight gain targets set by their doctor may be impossible to meet without occasionally being in ketosis. It's basic nutritional biochemistry, not a pathological state.

A Low Carbohydrate Diet Is the Original Prenatal Diet

The stunning rates of gestational diabetes have made some researchers question its purpose in pregnancy. We know from animal data that *all* mammals have physiological changes during pregnancy that facilitate increased insulin production and insulin resistance, which suggests that it is a normal and genetically programmed response.[132] It only becomes problematic when a woman is unable to maintain normal blood sugar, and hence gets the diagnosis of gestational diabetes.

In fact, insulin concentrations spike 3 to 3.5 fold by the 10th week of pregnancy in normal gestation and remain elevated until delivery.[132] In early pregnancy, insulin sensitivity remains the same, but in late pregnancy as the metabolism shifts to provide the rapidly growing baby with fuel, insulin sensitivity is reduced by 50-70%. Women in late pregnancy are also up to 30% more efficient at creating glucose from alternative sources (called gluconeogenesis), which questions the need for high levels of ingested glucose (from carbohydrates) to supply the fetus.[133]

Some hypothesize that these changes in insulin and metabolism have evolved as an adaptation to the dietary pattern humans were accustomed to thousands of years ago, before modern agriculture, which just so happened to be very low in carbohydrates.[132] If this is the case, insulin resistance would serve to reduce glucose use by the mother and instead shunt that glucose to the growing fetus. Because the human genome has not changed considerably in the past 10,000 years, perhaps this means humans are metabolically adapted to a low-carbohydrate diet during pregnancy.

Certainly hunter-gatherers had limited access to starchy foods, no access to refined sugars, and conceivably went periods of 12 hours or longer without eating, practically guaranteeing that they experienced ketosis during their pregnancies.

Data on ancestral diets indeed shows many cultures followed a low-carbohydrate diet before the introduction of industrialized agriculture. The Inuit and other Alaskan and Canadian native people seemingly reproduced without difficulty following their traditional diet, which was high in fat (mostly from animals), moderate in protein, and extremely limited in carbohydrates.[134]

While we can't guarantee one dietary pattern will work for all people, to arbitrarily set a minimum recommended level of carbohydrates for pregnancy when we have evidence of cultures reproducing successfully on lower carbohydrate intakes seems illogical.

Summary

The data presented above has given me enough reassurance to reduce my prenatal carbohydrate recommendations, as I have presented in this book. While it seems unlikely we'll ever have a randomized controlled trial on a prenatal diet providing less than 40% of calories from carbohydrates, I do hope that those trials are completed at some point. As you'll notice, I suggest a variable amount of carbohydrates ranging from 90-150 grams per day to allow for individualization based on prepregnancy weight, blood sugar, use of medications, and weight gain goals. I know many women who have had successful pregnancies at even lower carbohydrate levels.

Following these recommendations and with the emphasis I place on mindful eating, the majority of my clients are able to manage their blood sugar with minimal or no need for insulin and medication. Moreover, their energy levels stay stable, they avoid extreme hunger or fullness, they rarely, if ever, experience hypoglycemia or hyperglycemia, and their babies grow normally. I know many medical providers who secretly recommend dietary guidelines similar to those I present in this book, but few are willing to speak publicly about it. But I believe it's time we start questioning the status quo when it comes to prenatal diet.

If I can instill anything in you, it's this: You make the choices about your health care, food, and exercise. Whether or not you take my advice, I hope this section has given you a deeper understanding of how your metabolism changes during pregnancy and how you can use food to help you and your baby stay healthy.

Jennifer's Story

I've had gestational diabetes with each of my 6 pregnancies. With my first pregnancy, I followed everything my doctor told me and attended the nutrition class with the dietitian. My gestational diabetes was so severe that I had to take big doses of insulin with each meal. I developed preeclampsia and ended up being induced at 35 weeks because my blood pressure and blood sugar were out of control.

With my second through fifth pregnancies, I had similar difficulties.

But with my sixth pregnancy, I had a completely different experience. Before I got pregnant that time, I had started eating a low carb Paleo/Primal type diet and lost 55 pounds. And while I was still overweight, my A1c was 5.7% at the beginning of the pregnancy (it was over 6% after my prior pregnancy). By 37 weeks, I'd only gained 2 pounds and my son measured exactly on target at each visit.

The only blood sugar number I had trouble controlling was my fasting number. I tried just about everything to get that down to normal, from changing the time I exercised, trying different dinners or bedtime snacks, apple cider vinegar, cinnamon. You name it, I tried it. And I'm glad I tried all of that, because I learned a lot about my body. I ended up needing some NPH insulin at night to correct my fasting number, but all of my other blood sugar numbers were diet controlled. Actually, my average blood sugar (fasting and post meal numbers) was 95.

This was the first pregnancy where I didn't have the typical complaints. I had no swelling, I walked 3 miles every night and still had plenty of energy, I slept great and woke up energized, I worked full time even into my last month, and I manage a household of 5 kids and a husband. Also, my blood pressure was completely normal despite my history of preeclampsia. I believe the only way I could do it is because I didn't have the sugar highs and lows from eating too many carbohydrates.

The only thing I consciously looked at was carbohydrates and stayed around 65g per day. All my carbs came from veggies, fruit, nuts, and full-fat dairy products (no grains). I wouldn't necessarily recommend all women eat at this level of carbohydrates, but I know my body is highly insulin resistant and does better at a lower level.

The frustrating thing is I had to learn all of this myself, especially when it came to ketones. I still can't wrap my mind around the idea that doctors worry when a woman with gestational diabetes has ketones, but could care less about ketones in a woman with morning sickness. The biggest hurdle being pregnant and eating this way was managing the ketone argument with my doctor. I'd have to carb load the night before I went in for doctor visits, so ketones don't show up in my urine the next morning. Dealing with providers can be a major challenge when they don't understand that ketosis is a natural byproduct of pregnancy and is *not* the same thing as diabetic ketoacidosis.

In the end, I'm happy with my decision to eat low carb during this pregnancy. It certainly made my gestational diabetes easier to manage and my whole pregnancy was easy compared to my five others. I hope more women will be open to this once they understand the research behind this and I hope more doctors and nutritionists will be on board someday.

Appendix

Recipes

This section includes a selection of recipes from the meal plans included in Chapter 4. For even more gestational diabetes-friendly recipes, visit www.RealFoodforGD.com.

Breakfast Recipes

Crustless Spinach Quiche
Grain-free Granola

Lunch and Dinner Recipes

Beanless Beef Chili
Salmon Salad
Roasted Curried Cauliflower
Grass-fed Beef Meatloaf
Roasted Carrots, Celery, and Onions
Homemade Chicken Vegetable Soup
Homemade Chicken Stock (or bone broth)
Slow Cooker Carnitas
Tomato-Cream Sauce (to serve with spaghetti squash)
Grass-fed Beef Meatballs
Low-carb Shepherd's Pie
Coconut Chicken Curry

Snack and Dessert Recipes

Homemade Berry Sorbet
Coconut Macaroons
Nutty "Granola" Bars

Breakfast Recipes

Crustless Spinach Quiche

Makes 6 servings.

Ingredients

1 tablespoon coconut oil or butter
1 onion, chopped
10oz package frozen, chopped spinach, thawed and drained
5 eggs, ideally from pastured chickens
3 cups shredded cheese (Muenster, cheddar or jack)
1/2 teaspoon salt
1/8 teaspoon black pepper

Directions

In a large skillet, cook onions in coconut oil or butter until soft.
Stir in spinach and allow excess moisture to evaporate.
In a large bowl, mix eggs, cheese, salt, and pepper.
Add spinach-onion mixture and stir to combine.
Pour into a buttered 9-inch pie dish.
Bake in a 350 degree oven until eggs set, about 30 minutes.
Let cool for 15 minutes before serving.

NOTE: You may substitute any cooked green for the spinach, such as kale.

Grain-free Granola

Makes 10 servings (1/2 cup each)

Ingredients

¼ cup coconut oil or butter, melted
3 cups unsweetened coconut flakes
1 cup sliced almonds
1 cup chopped walnuts, pecans, hazelnuts, macadamia nuts (or combination)
2 tablespoons chia seeds, whole
2 tablespoons pure maple syrup
2 teaspoons ground cinnamon
¼ teaspoon ground nutmeg
1/2 teaspoon sea salt

Directions

Melt coconut oil or butter in a small saucepan.
Mix with remaining ingredients.
Spread onto a large baking sheet and bake for 25 minutes at 275 degrees until golden brown and fragrant. Be sure not to over-bake. Granola will crisp as it cools.
Store at room temperature in an airtight container for up to 1 month.

NOTE: You may add stevia to taste if you'd like a sweeter granola.

Lunch and Dinner Recipes

Beanless Beef Chili

Makes 6 servings

Ingredients

1 dried chipotle pepper, stem removed
1 cup boiling water
1 1/2 teaspoons coconut oil
1 cup chopped yellow onion
1 cup chopped green bell pepper
1 cup chopped red bell pepper
4 garlic cloves, minced
1 pound ground beef (grass-fed)
1/2 pound spicy ground pork sausage
1 tablespoon chili powder
1 tablespoon ground cumin
1 teaspoon dried oregano
1 teaspoon unsweetened cocoa powder
1 teaspoon Worcestershire sauce
1 (28 ounce) can crushed tomatoes
1 1/2 teaspoons sea salt
1/2 teaspoon ground black pepper

Directions

Soak chipotle pepper in boiling water until softened, about 10 minutes. Remove pepper from water and mince.
Melt coconut oil in a large pot over medium heat.
Add onion and bell peppers to the pan. Cook until tender, 5 to 10 minutes.
Stir garlic and minced chipotle into onion mixture and cook until fragrant, about 1 minute.
Add beef and sausage to the pan. Cook and stir until meat is browned and crumbly, 10 to 12 minutes.

Add remaining ingredients, stir to combine. Bring to a boil, reduce heat to low, and simmer until flavors are developed, 10 minutes.

NOTE: Chili often tastes better the next day. Make extra and consider freezing for quick meals.

Salmon Salad

Makes 3-4 servings

Ingredients

16 oz wild Alaskan salmon, cooked, skin and bones removed
(may use canned)
1 cup celery, finely diced
1/4 cup small-diced red onion (1 small onion)
1 tablespoon minced fresh dill
1 tablespoons capers, drained
1 tablespoons apple cider vinegar
1 tablespoons extra virgin olive oil
1/4 teaspoon sea salt (or more to taste)
1/4 teaspoon freshly ground black pepper

Directions

Place the salmon in a medium bowl.
Add remaining ingredients and gently mix to combine.
Serve cold or at room temperature.

NOTE: Salmon salad is excellent served over a salad, as a
lettuce wrap, or spread on vegetable slices, such as
cucumber, celery, and bell pepper.

Roasted Curried Cauliflower

Makes 6 servings

Ingredients

1 large head cauliflower, about 2 lbs, cut into small florets, roughly the same size
1 onion, sliced
1-2 inch knob fresh ginger, finely grated OR 1 teaspoon ground dried ginger
2-3 heaping tablespoons curry powder (If you don't like spicy, buy a mild curry powder)
2 cloves garlic, minced OR 1 teaspoon garlic powder
2 teaspoons sea salt, or more (Use approximately 1 teaspoon per pound of vegetables)
½ teaspoon freshly ground pepper
16 oz can coconut milk, full-fat
1-2 tablespoons coconut oil or ghee or butter (ghee is Indian clarified butter)
1 tablespoon balsamic vinegar or pomegranate molasses (Pomegranate molasses is found in Middle Eastern markets)

Directions

Cut up all vegetables and place on a large baking pan, such as a lasagne dish. You want a single layer, so if it's piled up, split it into 2 pans. The smaller the pieces, the faster it will cook.
Add all spices.
Pour in coconut milk, oil/ghee, and vinegar/pomegranate molasses. Mix.
Bake in preheated 425 degree oven for 30-40 min or until cauliflower is lightly browned and tender when pierced with a fork.
Serve hot or cold.

Grass-fed Beef Meatloaf

Makes 8 servings.

Ingredients

Meatloaf:
1 small onion, finely diced
8oz mushrooms, finely diced
2 cloves garlic, minced
2 tablespoons coconut oil
1 small zucchini, grated
2 lbs grass fed ground beef
6 ounces grass-fed beef liver, finely chopped or ground
2 eggs, ideally from pastured chickens
1/4 cup almond meal or coconut flour
2 teaspoons sea salt
1/2 teaspoon black pepper
1 teaspoon dried oregano
1 teaspoon dried thyme

Topping:
6 ounces tomato paste (1 small can)
1 tablespoon maple syrup or honey
1 packet stevia (optional, if you prefer this to be sweet, like ketchup)
1 teaspoon soy sauce

Directions

In a large skillet over medium-high heat, sauté onion, mushrooms, and garlic in coconut oil until lightly browned and all water (released from the vegetables) has evaporated from the skillet. Set aside to cool.
In a large mixing bowl, mix meat, cooked vegetables, and all remaining meatloaf ingredients.
Form into a loaf shape in a 9 x 13 inch glass baking dish.
Mix topping ingredients. Adjust seasonings to taste. Spoon

over meatloaf.

Bake meatloaf in a 350 degree oven for 45-60 minutes, or until cooked through.

NOTE: This recipe is a great way to include nutrient-dense liver in your diet if you're not a fan of the taste.

Roasted Carrots, Celery, and Onions

Makes 8 servings.

Ingredients

4 large carrots, peeled, diced
6 stalks celery, diced
1 large onion, diced
3 tablespoons coconut oil, melted
1 1/2 teaspoons sea salt
1/2 teaspoon black pepper
1 teaspoon dried thyme
1 teaspoon garlic powder

Directions

On a large baking pan (a half-sheet pan or lasagne dish is ideal), combine all ingredients.

Bake in a 400 degree oven for 30-45 minutes, turning occasionally, until vegetables are lightly brown and can be easily pierced with a fork.

Homemade Chicken Vegetable Soup

Makes 4 servings.

Ingredients

1 large onion, chopped
3 large carrots, peeled, chopped
4 stalks celery, chopped
2 tablespoons butter
1 teaspoon sea salt, or to taste
1/2 teaspoon black pepper
1/2 teaspoon dried thyme
4 cups (1 quart) chicken stock, ideally homemade*
1 lb chicken meat, picked from a roasted chicken (or pre-cooked chicken thigh meat, chopped)
1/2 cup heavy cream
1 tablespoon lemon juice
2 tablespoons fresh parsley, to garnish (optional)

Directions

In a large pot over high heat, sauté all vegetables in butter with salt, pepper, and thyme until lightly browned and fragrant.
Add chicken stock and bring to a boil.
Add chicken meat, heavy cream, and lemon juice. Reduce heat and simmer for 5 minutes.
Adjust seasonings to taste.
Serve with fresh parsley.

NOTE: *See Homemade Chicken Stock recipe.

Homemade Chicken Stock (or bone broth)

Ingredients

1 whole chicken or turkey -or- 2 to 3 pounds of bony parts, such as necks, backs, breastbones, wings, and feet (ideally from pastured birds)*
2 tablespoons vinegar or lemon juice (this helps leach more minerals from the bones)
1 large onion, skin on, cut into quarters
2-4 carrots, whole
2-4 celery stalks, ideally with leaves
1 bay leaf
½ teaspoon black peppercorns (optional)
vegetable scraps – (optionally add kale stems, parsley, garlic, ginger, etc)
cold filtered water, to cover

Directions

Place all ingredients in a large slow cooker or pot. Cover with water.
Bring to a simmer and cook on low for at least 24 hours.
Skim off impurities or "foam" and discard.
The stock is done when the bones are soft. The ends of chicken or turkey bones should literally crumble, otherwise you can let it continue cooking to maximize the mineral content of the broth. (Beef bones can be used for a second batch of stock.)
When finished, the stock should be a rich golden color.
Let cool, strain, and store in the refrigerator for up to 3 days or freeze for long-term storage.

*May substitute beef bones for beef stock.

TIP: Freeze leftover stock as ice cubes to defrost quickly!

Slow Cooker Carnitas

Makes 16 servings.

Ingredients

4-5 lb pork shoulder, ideally from a pasture-raised pig
1 onion, finely sliced
2 teaspoons sea salt
1 teaspoon garlic powder
1 teaspoon chili powder
1 teaspoon cumin
1 teaspoon oregano
juice of 2 limes (or 2 tablespoons apple cider vinegar)

Directions

Place onions in bottom of slow cooker.
Mix spices and salt. Rub over pork shoulder and place in the slow cooker.
Add lime juice or vinegar.
Cook on high for 6-8 hours.
When finished, the pork will easily shred with a fork. Adjust cooking time as necessary.
Remove pork and either eat as is -or- Place drained meat in a cast iron skillet with some rendered pork fat (there'll be a layer on top of your slow cooker). Cook on high heat until pork is crisp around the edges.
Serve and enjoy!

Tomato-Cream Sauce

Makes 10 servings.

Ingredients

2 tablespoons butter
2 tablespoons extra virgin olive oil
1 medium onion, chopped
1/2 teaspoon salt, to taste
1/2 teaspoon black pepper
1 teaspoon oregano
3 cloves garlic, minced
28 oz canned, chopped tomatoes
1 cup heavy cream
1/2 cup fresh basil leaves, torn into pieces

Directions

Heat the butter and oil in a large skillet over medium heat.
Add onions, salt, pepper, and oregano. Cook for 5 minutes.
Add the garlic and cook for another 2 minutes, being sure not to burn the garlic.
Add chopped tomatoes, reduce heat to low.
Cook for 25-30 minutes, stirring occasionally.
Remove the sauce from the heat and stir in the cream.
Check the seasoning and adjust as needed.
Add the chopped basil and serve over cooked spaghetti squash.

Grass-fed Beef Meatballs

Makes 4 servings.

Ingredients

1 small onion, finely diced
8 oz mushrooms, finely diced
2 cloves garlic, minced
2 tablespoons coconut oil
1 lb grass fed ground beef
3 ounces grass-fed beef liver, finely chopped or ground (optional)
1 egg, ideally from pastured chickens
1 teaspoon sea salt
1/4 teaspoon black pepper
1/2 teaspoon dried oregano

Directions

In a large skillet over medium-high heat, sauté onion, mushrooms, and garlic in coconut oil until lightly browned and all water (released from the vegetables) has evaporated from the skillet. Set aside to cool.
In a large mixing bowl, mix meat with cooked vegetables and remaining ingredients.
Form into 12 meatballs.
Place meatballs at least 1 inch apart on a greased baking dish.
Bake in a 350 degree oven for 15-20 minutes, or until cooked through.

NOTE: This recipe is a great way to include nutrient-dense liver in your diet if you're not a fan of the taste.

Low-carb Shepherd's Pie

Makes 6 servings.

Ingredients

Filling:
1 lb grass fed ground beef
3 ounces grass-fed beef liver, finely chopped (optional)
1 small onion, finely diced
3 carrots, peeled, finely diced
2 stalks celery, finely diced
2 cloves garlic, minced
1 tablespoon butter
1 teaspoon salt
½ teaspoon black pepper
2 teaspoons dried thyme

Cauliflower Topping:
1 large head cauliflower, chopped
4 tablespoons butter
1 teaspoon sea salt, or to taste
1/2 teaspoon black pepper

Directions

Steam cauliflower while preparing the filling, which takes 10-15 minutes, depending on the size of cauliflower pieces.
In a large skillet, cook ground beef over medium-high heat. If the pan is dry, add a bit of butter or coconut oil (grass-fed beef can be very lean).
With a spatula, break up meat into bite-sized pieces. Once browned, add liver and cook for 1-2 minutes.
Remove from heat and place in a 9x13 inch baking dish. *Do not* drain rendered fat.
In the same pan, add butter, onion, carrots, celery, garlic, salt, pepper, and thyme.
Cook for 10 minutes, being sure to scrape up browned bits.

Mash steamed cauliflower with butter, salt, and pepper. Spread on top of meat and vegetables.
Bake in a 400 degree oven for 20 minutes, until cauliflower is lightly browned.

NOTE: This recipe is a great way to include nutrient-dense liver in your diet if you're not a fan of the taste.

Coconut Chicken Curry

Makes 8 servings.

Ingredients

1 medium onion, finely diced
1 cup fresh green beans, trimmed, cut into 2 inch pieces
1 green bell pepper, thinly sliced
1 red bell pepper, thinly sliced
2 cloves garlic, minced
2 tablespoons freshly grated ginger
1 tablespoon coconut oil
2 tablespoons mild curry powder (such as garam masala)
1 teaspoon sea salt
15 oz full-fat coconut milk
16 oz chicken broth (ideally homemade)
16 oz cooked, shredded chicken
Handful of fresh spinach
juice of 2 limes
dash of soy sauce or tamari, to taste
chili flakes or fresh chili slices (optional)

Directions

In a medium pot over medium-high heat, sauté onion in coconut oil until lightly browned.
Add all remaining vegetables, garlic, ginger, curry powder, and salt. Cook for 5 minutes.
Add coconut milk, broth, and chicken.
Simmer for 10 minutes.
Add lime and tamari to taste.
Just before serving, add fresh spinach and stir to wilt.

Snack and Dessert Recipes

Homemade Berry Sorbet

Makes 2 servings.

Ingredients

1 cup frozen berries (blueberries, raspberries, or blackberries)
1/2 cup heavy whipping cream
1 tablespoon powdered gelatin or collagen* (optional)
1 packet stevia sweetener or 5-10 drops liquid stevia extract (optional)

Directions

Puree all ingredients using a blender, immersion blender, or food processor.
Serve immediately.

* Great Lakes brand is made from grass-fed beef. Their product, "Hydrolyzed Collagen", is ideal for this recipe, because it dissolves completely in cold liquids. This provides a nourishing source of protein and glycine to this recipe, but is not required.

Coconut Macaroons

Makes 36 cookies.

Ingredients

5 egg whites*
1/4 teaspoon sea salt
1/3 cup honey
1 tablespoon vanilla extract (or almond extract)
3 cups shredded coconut, <u>unsweetened</u>

Directions

In a large bowl, whisk egg whites and salt until stiff.
Fold in remaining ingredients.
With a spoon, scoop out 1 tablespoon portions and drop onto a parchment-lined baking sheet.
Bake at 350 degrees for 10-15 minutes, until lightly browned.

* Save the egg yolks for scrambled eggs, mixing into meatloaf/meatballs, or another recipe. They are too good to throw away!

Nutty "Granola" Bars

Ingredients

4 tablespoons ground flaxseeds or chia seeds
1/2 cup raw honey
1 egg
1 teaspoon sea salt
1 cup raw almonds pieces
1 cup raw walnuts pieces (or other nuts)
1 cup unsweetened large coconut flakes
1 cup unsweetened fine coconut flakes

Directions

Mix the ground flaxseeds or chia seeds with honey in a small bowl.
In a large bowl, mix remaining ingredients.
Add honey mixture to large bowl, stirring to combine.
Line a sheet tray with parchment paper and scoop mix onto paper.
Lay another piece of parchment paper on top of the mixture and with your hands spread it evenly on tray so that it extends all the way to the sides.
Press the mixture down firmly with a flat surface, like the bottom of a small pot.
Remove top layer of parchment paper and place in 350 degree oven.
Bake for 24 minutes, rotating the tray at 12 minutes.
Let cool and cut into 24 bars.

For more gestational diabetes-friendly recipes, visit www.RealFoodforGD.com.

References

1 Kim, Catherine, Katherine M Newton, and Robert H Knopp. "Gestational Diabetes and the Incidence of Type 2 Diabetes A systematic review." Diabetes Care 25.10 (2002): 1862-1868.

2 Coustan, Donald R et al. "The Hyperglycemia and Adverse Pregnancy Outcome (HAPO) study: paving the way for new diagnostic criteria for gestational diabetes mellitus." American Journal of Obstetrics and Gynecology 202.6 (2010): 654. e1-654. e6.

3 Kim, Shin Y et al. "Racial/ethnic differences in the percentage of gestational diabetes mellitus cases attributable to overweight and obesity, Florida, 2004-2007." Preventing Chronic Disease 9 (2012).

4 Coustan, Donald, et al. "Maternal age and screening for gestational diabetes: a population-based study." Obstetrics & Gynecology 73.4 (1989): 557-561.

5 Holder, Tara et al. "A low disposition index in adolescent offspring of mothers with gestational diabetes: a risk marker for the development of impaired glucose tolerance in youth." Diabetologia 57.11 (2014): 2413-2420.

6 Hernandez, Teri L et al. "Patterns of Glycemia in Normal Pregnancy Should the current therapeutic targets be challenged?." Diabetes Care 34.7 (2011): 1660-1668.

7 Miller, Carla K et al. "Comparative effectiveness of a mindful eating intervention to a diabetes self-management intervention among adults with type 2 diabetes: a pilot study." Journal of the Academy of Nutrition and Dietetics 112.11 (2012): 1835-1842.

8 Yang, Qing. "Gain weight by "going diet?" Artificial sweeteners and the neurobiology of sugar cravings: Neuroscience 2010." The Yale Journal of Biology and Medicine 83.2 (2010): 101.

9 Suez, Jotham et al. "Artificial sweeteners induce glucose intolerance by altering the gut microbiota." Nature 514.7521 (2014): 181-186.

10 Abou-Donia, Mohamed B et al. "Splenda alters gut microflora and increases intestinal p-glycoprotein and cytochrome p-450 in male rats." Journal of Toxicology and Environmental Health, Part A 71.21 (2008): 1415-1429.

11 Morrison, John A, Charles J Glueck, and Ping Wang. "Dietary trans fatty acid intake is associated with increased fetal loss." Fertility and Sterility 90.2 (2008): 385-390.

12 Karsten, HD et al. "Vitamins A, E and fatty acid composition of the eggs of caged hens and pastured hens." Renewable Agriculture and Food Systems 25.01 (2010): 45-54.

13 Shaw, Gary M et al. "Periconceptional dietary intake of choline and betaine and neural tube defects in offspring." American Journal of Epidemiology 160.2 (2004): 102-109.

14 Jiang, Xinyin et al. "Maternal choline intake alters the epigenetic state of fetal cortisol-regulating genes in humans." The FASEB Journal 26.8 (2012): 3563-3574.

15 Zeisel, Steven H. "Nutritional importance of choline for brain development." Journal of the American College of Nutrition 23.sup6 (2004): 621S-626S.

16 Jensen, Helen H et al. "Choline in the diets of the US population: NHANES, 2003–2004." FASEB J 21 (2007): lb219.

17 West, Allyson A et al. "Choline intake influences phosphatidylcholine DHA enrichment in nonpregnant women but not in pregnant women in the third trimester." American Journal of Clinical Nutrition 97.4 (2013): 718-727.

18 Ratliff, Joseph et al. "Consuming eggs for breakfast influences plasma glucose and ghrelin, while reducing energy intake during the next 24 hours in adult men." Nutrition Research 30.2 (2010): 96-103.

19 Fernandez, Maria Luz, and Mariana Calle. "Revisiting dietary cholesterol recommendations: does the evidence support a limit of 300 mg/d?." Current Atherosclerosis Reports 12.6 (2010): 377-383.

20 Volek, Jeff S et al. "Carbohydrate restriction has a more favorable impact on the metabolic syndrome than a low fat diet." Lipids 44.4 (2009): 297-309.

21 Centers for Disease Control and Prevention (CDC). Surveillance for Foodborne Disease Outbreaks, United States, 2012, Annual Report. Atlanta, Georgia: US Department of Health and Human Services, CDC, 2014.

22 Alali, Walid Q et al. "Prevalence and distribution of Salmonella in organic and conventional broiler poultry farms." Foodborne pathogens and disease 7.11 (2010): 1363-1371.

23 Molloy, Anne M et al. "Effects of folate and vitamin B12 deficiencies during pregnancy on fetal, infant, and child development." Food & Nutrition Bulletin 29.Supplement 1 (2008): 101-111.

24 Masterjohn, Christopher. "Vitamin D toxicity redefined: vitamin K and the molecular mechanism." Medical Hypotheses 68.5 (2007): 1026-1034.

25 Buss, NE et al. "The teratogenic metabolites of vitamin A in women following supplements and liver." Human & Experimental Toxicology 13.1 (1994): 33-43.

26 Strobel, Manuela, Jana Tinz, and Hans-Konrad Biesalski. "The importance of β-carotene as a source of vitamin A with special regard to pregnant and breastfeeding women." European Journal of Nutrition 46.9 (2007): 1-20.

27 Harrison, Earl H. "Mechanisms involved in the intestinal absorption of dietary vitamin A and provitamin A carotenoids." Biochimica et Biophysica Acta (BBA)-Molecular and Cell Biology of Lipids 1821.1 (2012): 70-77.

28 Tang, Guangwen. "Bioconversion of dietary provitamin A carotenoids to vitamin A in humans." The American Journal of Clinical Nutrition 91.5 (2010): 1468S-1473S.

29 Novotny, Janet A et al. "β-Carotene conversion to vitamin A decreases as the dietary dose increases in humans." The Journal of Nutrition 140.5 (2010): 915-918.

30 Rees, William D, Fiona A Wilson, and Christopher A Maloney. "Sulfur amino acid metabolism in pregnancy: the impact of methionine in the maternal diet." The Journal of Nutrition 136.6 (2006): 1701S-1705S.

31 Persaud, Chandarika et al. "The excretion of 5☐oxoproline in urine, as an index of glycine status, during normal pregnancy." BJOG: An International Journal of Obstetrics & Gynaecology 96.4 (1989): 440-444.

32 Dasarathy, Jaividhya et al. "Methionine metabolism in human pregnancy." The American Journal of Clinical Nutrition 91.2 (2010): 357-365.

33 Friesen, Russell W et al. "Relationship of dimethylglycine, choline, and betaine with oxoproline in plasma of pregnant women and their newborn infants." The Journal of Nutrition 137.12 (2007): 2641-2646.

34 Rees, William D. "Manipulating the sulfur amino acid content of the early diet and its implications for long-term health." Proceedings of the Nutrition Society 61.01 (2002): 71-77.

35 Morrione, Thomas G, and Sam Seifter. "Alteration in the collagen content of the human uterus during pregnancy and post partum involution." The Journal of Experimental Medicine 115.2 (1962): 357-365.

36 Brown, Melody J et al. "Carotenoid bioavailability is higher from salads ingested with full-fat than with fat-reduced salad dressings as measured with electrochemical detection." The American Journal of Clinical Nutrition 80.2 (2004): 396-403.

37 Ralston, Nicholas VC, and Laura J Raymond. "Dietary selenium's protective effects against methylmercury toxicity." Toxicology 278.1 (2010): 112-123.

38 Burger, Joanna, and Michael Gochfeld. "Mercury and selenium levels in 19 species of saltwater fish from New Jersey as a function of species, size, and season." Science of the Total Environment 409.8 (2011): 1418-1429.

39 Bodnar, Lisa M et al. "High prevalence of vitamin D insufficiency in black and white pregnant women residing in the northern United States and their neonates." The Journal of Nutrition 137.2 (2007): 447-452.

40 Zimmermann, Michael B. "The effects of iodine deficiency in pregnancy and infancy." Paediatric and Perinatal Epidemiology 26.s1 (2012): 108-117.

41 Stagnaro-Green, Alex, Scott Sullivan, and Elizabeth N Pearce. "Iodine supplementation during pregnancy and lactation." JAMA 308.23 (2012): 2463-2464.

42 Mozaffarian, Dariush, and Eric B Rimm. "Fish intake, contaminants, and human health: evaluating the risks and the benefits." JAMA 296.15 (2006): 1885-1899.

43 Tsuchie, Hiroyuki et al. "Amelioration of pregnancy-associated osteoporosis after treatment with vitamin K2: a report of four patients." Upsala Journal of Medical Sciences 117.3 (2012): 336-341.

44 Choi, Hyung Jin et al. "Vitamin K2 supplementation improves insulin sensitivity via osteocalcin metabolism: a placebo-controlled trial." Diabetes Care 34.9 (2011): e147-e147.

45 Bertelsen, Randi J et al. "Probiotic milk consumption in pregnancy and infancy and subsequent childhood allergic diseases." Journal of Allergy and Clinical Immunology 133.1 (2014): 165-171. e8.

46 Myhre, Ronny et al. "Intake of probiotic food and risk of spontaneous preterm delivery." The American Journal of Clinical Nutrition 93.1 (2011): 151-157.

47 Greenberg, James A, and Stacey J Bell. "Multivitamin supplementation during pregnancy: emphasis on folic acid and L-methylfolate." Reviews in Obstetrics and Gynecology 4.3-4 (2011): 126.

48 Schmid, Alexandra, and Barbara Walther. "Natural vitamin D content in animal products." Advances in Nutrition: An International Review Journal 4.4 (2013): 453-462.

49 Bodnar, Lisa M et al. "High prevalence of vitamin D insufficiency in black and white pregnant women residing in the northern United States and their neonates." The Journal of Nutrition 137.2 (2007): 447-452.

50 Dawodu, Adekunle, and Reginald C Tsang. "Maternal vitamin D status: effect on milk vitamin D content and vitamin D status of breastfeeding infants." Advances in Nutrition: An International Review Journal 3.3 (2012): 353-361.

51 Lee, Joyce M et al. "Vitamin D deficiency in a healthy group of mothers and newborn infants." Clinical Pediatrics 46.1 (2007): 42-44.

52 Viljakainen, HT et al. "Maternal vitamin D status determines bone variables in the newborn." The Journal of Clinical Endocrinology & Metabolism 95.4 (2010): 1749-1757.

53 Wei, Shu-Qin et al. "Maternal vitamin D status and adverse pregnancy outcomes: a systematic review and meta-analysis." The Journal of Maternal-Fetal & Neonatal Medicine 26.9 (2013): 889-899.

54 Aghajafari, Fariba et al. "Association between maternal serum 25-hydroxyvitamin D level and pregnancy and neonatal outcomes: systematic review and meta-analysis of observational studies." BMJ: British Medical Journal 346 (2013).

55 Zhang, Cuilin et al. "Maternal plasma 25-hydroxyvitamin D concentrations and the risk for gestational diabetes mellitus." PLoS One 3.11 (2008): e3753.

56 Lau, Sue Lynn et al. "Serum 25-hydroxyvitamin D and glycated haemoglobin levels in women with gestational diabetes mellitus." Med J Aust 194.7 (2011): 334-337.

57 Nozza, Josephine M, and Christine P Rodda. "Vitamin D deficiency in mothers of infants with rickets." The Medical Journal of Australia 175.5 (2001): 253-255.

58 Javaid, MK et al. "Maternal vitamin D status during pregnancy and childhood bone mass at age 9 years: a longitudinal study." The Lancet 367.9504 (2006): 36-43.

59 Litonjua, Augusto A. "Childhood asthma may be a consequence of vitamin D deficiency." Current Opinion in Allergy and Clinical Immunology 9.3 (2009): 202.

60 Brehm, John M et al. "Serum vitamin D levels and markers of severity of childhood asthma in Costa Rica." American Journal of Respiratory and Critical Care Medicine 179.9 (2009): 765-771.

61 Whitehouse, Andrew JO et al. "Maternal serum vitamin D levels during pregnancy and offspring neurocognitive development." Pediatrics 129.3 (2012): 485-493.

62 Kinney, Dennis K et al. "Relation of schizophrenia prevalence to latitude, climate, fish consumption, infant mortality, and skin color: a role for prenatal vitamin d deficiency and infections?." Schizophrenia Bulletin (2009): sbp023.

63 Stene, LC et al. "Use of cod liver oil during pregnancy associated with lower risk of Type I diabetes in the offspring." Diabetologia 43.9 (2000): 1093-1098.

64 Salzer, Jonatan, Anders Svenningsson, and Peter Sundström. "Season of birth and multiple sclerosis in Sweden." Acta Neurologica Scandinavica 121.1 (2010): 20-23.

65 Hollis, Bruce W et al. "Vitamin D supplementation during pregnancy: Double□blind, randomized clinical trial of safety and effectiveness." Journal of Bone and Mineral Research 26.10 (2011): 2341-2357.

66 ACOG Committee on Obstetric Practice. "ACOG Committee Opinion No. 495: Vitamin D: Screening and supplementation during pregnancy." Obstetrics and Gynecology 118.1 (2011): 197.

67 Gerster, H. "Can adults adequately convert alpha-linoleni acid (18: 3n-3) to eicosapentaenoic acid (20: 5n-3) and docosahexaenoic acid (22: 6n-3)?." International Journal for Vitamin & Nutrition Research. 68.3 (1997):159-173.

68 Innis, Sheila M. "Dietary (n-3) fatty acids and brain development." The Journal of Nutrition 137.4 (2007): 855-859.

69 Aagaard, Kjersti et al. "The placenta harbors a unique microbiome." Science Translational Medicine 6.237 (2014): 237ra65-237ra65.

70 Mueller, Noel T et al. "Prenatal exposure to antibiotics, cesarean section and risk of childhood obesity." International Journal of Obesity (2014).

71 Luoto, Raakel et al. "Impact of maternal probiotic-supplemented dietary counselling on pregnancy outcome and prenatal and postnatal growth: a double-blind, placebo-controlled study." British Journal of Nutrition 103.12 (2010): 1792-1799.

72 Thoma, Marie E et al. "Bacterial vaginosis is associated with variation in dietary indices." The Journal of Nutrition 141.9 (2011): 1698-1704.

73 Bailey, Regan L et al. "Estimation of total usual calcium and vitamin D intakes in the United States." The Journal of Nutrition 140.4 (2010): 817-822.

74 Rosanoff, Andrea, Connie M Weaver, and Robert K Rude. "Suboptimal magnesium status in the United States: are the health consequences underestimated?." Nutrition Reviews 70.3 (2012): 153-164.

75 Bardicef, Mordechai et al. "Extracellular and intracellular magnesium depletion in pregnancy and gestational diabetes." American Journal of Obstetrics and Gynecology 172.3 (1995): 1009-1013.

76 Song, Yiqing et al. "Dietary magnesium intake in relation to plasma insulin levels and risk of type 2 diabetes in women." Diabetes Care 27.1 (2004): 59-65.

77 Mäder, Paul et al. "Soil fertility and biodiversity in organic farming." Science 296.5573 (2002): 1694-1697.

78 Evenson, Kelly R, A Savitz, and Sara L Huston. "Leisure□time physical activity among pregnant women in the US." Paediatric and Perinatal Epidemiology 18.6 (2004): 400-407.

79 Downs, Danielle Symons, and Jan S Ulbrecht. "Understanding exercise beliefs and behaviors in women with gestational diabetes mellitus." Diabetes Care 29.2 (2006): 236-240.

80 Collings, CA, LB Curet, and JP Mullin. "Maternal and fetal responses to a maternal aerobic exercise program." American Journal of Obstetrics and Gynecology 145.6 (1983): 702-707.

81 Melzer, Katarina et al. "Physical activity and pregnancy." Sports Medicine 40.6 (2010): 493-507.

82 Dempsey, Jennifer C et al. "A case-control study of maternal recreational physical activity and risk of gestational diabetes mellitus." Diabetes Research and Clinical Practice 66.2 (2004): 203-215.

83 Hillman, Charles H, Kirk I Erickson, and Arthur F Kramer. "Be smart, exercise your heart: exercise effects on brain and cognition." Nature Reviews Neuroscience 9.1 (2008): 58-65.

84 Jovanovic-Peterson, Lois, Eric P Durak, and Charles M Peterson. "Randomized trial of diet versus diet plus cardiovascular conditioning on glucose levels in gestational diabetes." American Journal of Obstetrics and Gynecology 161.2 (1989): 415-419.

85 Artal, Raul et al. "A lifestyle intervention of weight-gain restriction: diet and exercise in obese women with gestational diabetes mellitus." Applied Physiology, Nutrition, and Metabolism 32.3 (2007): 596-601.

86 Dempsey, Jennifer C et al. "A case-control study of maternal recreational physical activity and risk of gestational diabetes mellitus." Diabetes Research and Clinical Practice 66.2 (2004): 203-215.

87 Brenner, IK et al. "Physical conditioning effects on fetal heart rate responses to graded maternal exercise." Medicine and Science in Sports and Exercise 31.6 (1999): 792-799.

88 Hammer, Roger L, Jan Perkins, and Richard Parr. "Exercise during the childbearing year." The Journal of Perinatal Education 9.1 (2000): 1.

89 Moses, Robert G et al. "Can a low–glycemic index diet reduce the need for insulin in gestational diabetes mellitus? A randomized trial." Diabetes Care 32.6 (2009): 996-1000.

90 HAPO Study Cooperative Research Group. "Hyperglycemia and Adverse Pregnancy outcome (HAPO) study Associations with neonatal anthropometrics." Diabetes 58.2 (2009): 453-459.

91 Tertti, K et al. "Metformin vs. insulin in gestational diabetes. A randomized study characterizing metformin patients needing additional insulin." Diabetes, Obesity and Metabolism 15.3 (2013): 246-251.

92 Marques, Pedro et al. "Metformin safety in the management of gestational diabetes." Endocrine Practice (2014): 1-21.

93 Hague, WM et al. "Metformin crosses the placenta: A modulator for fetal insulin resistance?." British Medical Journal 327 (2004): 880-881.

94 Bauman, WILLIAM A et al. "Increased intake of calcium reverses vitamin B12 malabsorption induced by metformin." Diabetes Care 23.9 (2000): 1227-1231.

95 Aston-Mourney, K et al. "Too much of a good thing: why it is bad to stimulate the beta cell to secrete insulin." Diabetologia 51.4 (2008): 540-545.

96 Langer, Oded et al. "A comparison of glyburide and insulin in women with gestational diabetes mellitus." New England Journal of Medicine 343.16 (2000): 1134-1138.

97 HAPO Study Cooperative Research Group. "Hyperglycemia and Adverse Pregnancy Outcome (HAPO) study: associations with neonatal anthropometrics." Diabetes 58.2 (2009): 453-459.

98 McManus, Ruth M et al. "Beta-cell function and visceral fat in lactating women with a history of gestational diabetes." Metabolism 50.6 (2001): 715-719.

99 Kjos, Siri L et al. "The effect of lactation on glucose and lipid metabolism in women with recent gestational diabetes." Obstetrics & Gynecology 82.3 (1993): 451-455.

100 Liu, Bette, Louisa Jorm, and Emily Banks. "Parity, breastfeeding, and the subsequent risk of maternal type 2 diabetes." Diabetes Care 33.6 (2010): 1239-1241.

101 Crume, TL et al. "The impact of neonatal breast-feeding on growth trajectories of youth exposed and unexposed to diabetes in utero: the EPOCH Study." International Journal of Obesity 36.4 (2012): 529-534.

102 Dawodu, Adekunle, and Reginald C Tsang. "Maternal vitamin D status: effect on milk vitamin D content and vitamin D status of breastfeeding infants." Advances in Nutrition: An International Review Journal 3.3 (2012): 353-361.

103 Hollis, Bruce W, and Carol L Wagner. "Vitamin D requirements during lactation: high-dose maternal supplementation as therapy to prevent hypovitaminosis D for both the mother and the nursing infant." The American Journal of Clinical Nutrition 80.6 (2004): 1752S-1758S.

104 Ilcol, Yeşim Ozarda et al. "Choline status in newborns, infants, children, breast-feeding women, breast-fed infants and human breast milk." The Journal of Nutritional Biochemistry 16.8 (2005): 489-499.

105 Diabetes Prevention Program Research Group. "10-year follow-up of diabetes incidence and weight loss in the Diabetes Prevention Program Outcomes Study." The Lancet 374.9702 (2009): 1677-1686.

106 Bellamy, Leanne et al. "Type 2 diabetes mellitus after gestational diabetes: a systematic review and meta-analysis." The Lancet 373.9677 (2009): 1773-1779.

107 Kim, Catherine, Diana K Berger, and Shadi Chamany. "Recurrence of gestational diabetes mellitus a systematic review." Diabetes Care 30.5 (2007): 1314-1319.

108 Hughes, Ruth CE et al. "An Early Pregnancy HbA1c≥ 5.9%(41 mmol/mol) Is Optimal for Detecting Diabetes and Identifies Women at Increased Risk of Adverse Pregnancy Outcomes." Diabetes Care (2014): DC_141312.

109 Zhang, Cuilin et al. "Adherence to healthy lifestyle and risk of gestational diabetes mellitus: prospective cohort study." BMJ 349 (2014): g5450.

110 Dempsey, Jennifer C et al. "A case-control study of maternal recreational physical activity and risk of gestational diabetes mellitus." Diabetes Research and Clinical Practice 66.2 (2004): 203-215.

111 Luoto, Raakel et al. "Impact of maternal probiotic-supplemented dietary counselling on pregnancy outcome and prenatal and postnatal growth: a double-blind, placebo-controlled study." British Journal of Nutrition 103.12 (2010): 1792-1799.

112 Kremer, Carrie J, and Patrick Duff. "Glyburide for the treatment of gestational diabetes." American Journal of Obstetrics and Gynecology 190.5 (2004): 1438-1439.

113 Moses, Robert G et al. "Can a low–glycemic index diet reduce the need for insulin in gestational diabetes mellitus? A randomized trial." Diabetes Care 32.6 (2009): 996-1000.

114 Institute of Medicine (US). Panel on Macronutrients, and Institute of Medicine (US). Standing Committee on the Scientific Evaluation of Dietary Reference Intakes. Dietary Reference Intakes for energy, carbohydrate, fiber, fat, fatty acids, cholesterol, protein, and amino acids. Natl Academy Pr, 2005. pg 275-277.

115 Rizzo, Thomas A et al. "Prenatal and perinatal influences on long-term psychomotor development in offspring of diabetic mothers." American Journal of Obstetrics and Gynecology 173.6 (1995): 1753-1758.

116 Metzger, BoydE et al. "" Accelerated starvation" and the skipped breakfast in late normal pregnancy." The Lancet 319.8272 (1982): 588-592.

117 Felig, Philip, and Vincent Lynch. "Starvation in human pregnancy: hypoglycemia, hypoinsulinemia, and hyperketonemia." Science 170.3961 (1970): 990-992.

118 Herrera, E. "Metabolic adaptations in pregnancy and their implications for the availability of substrates to the fetus." European Journal of Clinical Nutrition 54 (2000): S47-51.

119 Coetzee, EJ, WPU Jackson, and PA Berman. "Ketonuria in pregnancy—with special reference to calorie-restricted food intake in obese diabetics." Diabetes 29.3 (1980): 177-181.

120 Huckabee, William E. "Abnormal resting blood lactate: I. The significance of hyperlactatemia in hospitalized patients." The American Journal of Medicine 30.6 (1961): 833-839.

121 Felig, Philip et al. "Amino acid metabolism during starvation in human pregnancy." Journal of Clinical Investigation 51.5 (1972): 1195.

122 Feinman, Richard David et al. "Dietary Carbohydrate restriction as the first approach in diabetes management. Critical review and evidence base." Nutrition (2014).

123 Churchill, JA, HW Berendes, and J Nemore. "Neuropsychological deficits in children of diabetic mothers." American Journal of Obstetrics and Gynecology 105.2 (1969): 257.

124 Freinkel, N et al. "The 1986 McCollum award lecture. Fuel-mediated teratogenesis during early organogenesis: the effects of increased concentrations of glucose, ketones, or somatomedin inhibitor during rat embryo culture." The American Journal of Clinical Nutrition 44.6 (1986): 986-995.

125 Manninen, Anssi H. "Metabolic effects of the very-low-carbohydrate diets: Misunderstood "villains" of human metabolism." J Int Soc Sports Nutr 1.2 (2004): 7-11.

126 Kraus, H., and Stumpf, B.: Interrelationship of glucose and ketone body metabolism in brain during early infancy. Regulatory role of pyruvate dehydrogenase. Biochemical and Clinical Aspects of Ketone Body Metabolism. Soling, H-D, and Seufert, C-D., Eds. Stuttgart, George Thieme Publishers, 1978, pp. 233-41.

127 Bougneres, PF et al. "Ketone body transport in the human neonate and infant." Journal of Clinical Investigation 77.1 (1986): 42.

128 Bon, C et al. "[Feto-maternal metabolism in human normal pregnancies: study of 73 cases]." Annales de Biologie Clinique Dec. 2006: 609-619.

129 Kiel, Deborah W et al. "Gestational weight gain and pregnancy outcomes in obese women: how much is enough?." Obstetrics & Gynecology 110.4 (2007): 752-758.

130 Hernandez, Teri L et al. "Patterns of Glycemia in Normal Pregnancy Should the current therapeutic targets be challenged?." Diabetes Care 34.7 (2011): 1660-1668.

131 Hedderson, Monique M et al. "Pregnancy weight gain and risk of neonatal complications: macrosomia, hypoglycemia, and hyperbilirubinemia." Obstetrics & Gynecology 108.5 (2006): 1153-1161.

132 Kopp, Wolfgang. "Role of high-insulinogenic nutrition in the etiology of gestational diabetes mellitus." Medical Hypotheses 64.1 (2005): 101-103.

133 Butte, Nancy F. "Carbohydrate and lipid metabolism in pregnancy: normal compared with gestational diabetes mellitus." The American Journal of Clinical Nutrition 71.5 (2000): 1256s-1261s.

134 Draper, Harold H. "The aboriginal Eskimo diet in modern perspective." American Anthropologist 79.2 (1977): 309-316.

About the Author

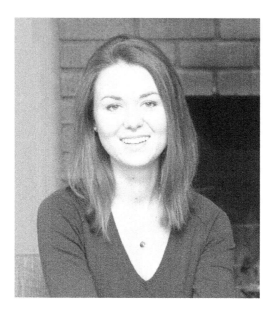

Lily Nichols is a Registered Dietitian/Nutritionist, Certified Diabetes Educator, Certified LEAP Therapist and Certified Pilates Instructor whose approach to nutrition embraces real food, integrative medicine, and mindful eating. Her fascination with the dietary practices of traditional cultures combined with an abnormal love for medical research, especially regarding prenatal nutrition, has led her to become one of the country's most sought after 'real food for pregnancy' experts. Lily has worked at the public policy level with the California Diabetes and Pregnancy Program: Sweet Success to update the nutritional and exercise guidelines for care as it relates to gestational diabetes, worked clinically with hundreds of women with gestational diabetes, and has helped train thousands of medical professionals on the subject of diabetes during pregnancy. Lily is also a regular speaker on a wide range of topics relating to prenatal nutrition and exercise.

182

Made in the USA
Middletown, DE
12 February 2021

33655140R00106